Dr. Robert L. Galli, MD
Professor and Chairman
Department of Emergency Medicine
University of Mississippi Medical Center
Jackson, Mississippi

Bold and innovative leaders, gifted educators, wise mentors, tireless workers, and talented clinicians come and go. They are to be found at every institution. What is extraordinarily rare is the individual who is all of these things and yet armed with a caring heart and sincere interest in all whom he meets, whether patient or peer. Thank you for all of these qualities and for always leading from the front.

Acknowledgments
My deepest gratitude to my parents, for showing the way; my wife, for her encouragement and tolerance of my moods; my daughter, for being the gift that she is.

Special thanks to
Dr. Robert Galli for his time, support, and leadership; Ms. Danay Trest and Ms. Melanie Hataway for their superb administrative skills and for dealing with my terrible handwriting.

WJP

Pain Management and Procedural Sedation Handbook

W. James Phillips, MD
Associate Professor of Anesthesia
Assistant Professor of Emergency Medicine
University of Mississippi Medical Center
Jackson, Mississippi

John Keith, MD
Assistant Professor of Emergency Medicine
University of Mississippi Medical Center
Jackson, Mississippi

Anna Lerant, MD
Associate Professor of Anesthesiology
University of Mississippi Medical Center
Jackson, Mississippi

Loretta Jackson Williams, MD, PhD
Associate Professor of Emergency Medicine
University of Mississippi Medical Center
Jackson, Mississippi

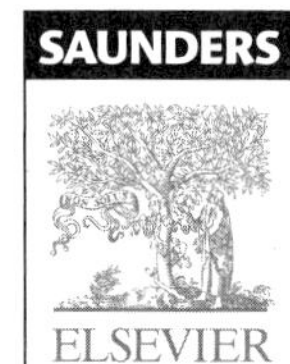

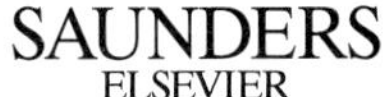

1600 John F. Kennedy Blvd.
Ste 1800
Philadelphia, PA 19103-2899

PAIN MANAGEMENT AND PROCEDURAL   978-0-323-05333-4
SEDATION HANDBOOK

Notice

Knowledge and best practice in this field are constantly changing. As new research and experience broaden our knowledge, changes in practice, treatment, and drug therapy may become necessary or appropriate. Readers are advised to check the most current information provided (i) on procedures featured or (ii) by the manufacturer of each product to be administered, to verify the recommended dose or formula, the method and duration of administration, and contraindications. It is the responsibility of the practitioner, relying on his or her experience and knowledge of the patient, to make diagnoses, to determine dosages and the best treatment for each individual patient, and to take all appropriate safety precautions. To the fullest extent of the law, neither the Publisher nor the Authors assume any liability for any injury and/or damage to persons or property arising out of or related to any use of the material contained in this book.

Library of Congress Cataloging-in-Publication Data

Pain management and procedural sedation handbook / W. James Phillips ... [et al.]. — 1st ed.
    p. ; cm.
  Includes bibliographical references.
  ISBN 978-0-323-05333-4
1. Pain—Treatment—Handbooks, manuals, etc. 2. Anesthesia—Handbooks, manuals, etc.
3. Analgesics—Handbooks, manuals. etc.   I. Phillips, W. James (William James)
  [DNLM: 1. Pain—therapy—Handbooks. 2. Analgesia—methods—Handbooks.
3. Analgesics—therapeutic use—Handbooks. WL 704 P145577 2008]

RB127.P3323416 2008
616'.0472—dc22   2007037184

Acquisitions Editor: James Merritt
Developmental Editor: Andrea Vosburgh
Publishing Services Manager: Linda Van Pelt
Project Manager: Sharon Lee
Design Direction: Ellen Zanolle

Working together to grow
libraries in developing countries

www.elsevier.com | www.bookaid.org | www.sabre.org

ELSEVIER   BOOK AID International   Sabre Foundation

Printed in the United States of America

Last digit is the print number: 9 8 7 6 5 4 3 2 1

Contributors

W. James Phillips, MD
Associate Professor of Anesthesia
Assistant Professor of Emergency Medicine
University of Mississippi Medical Center
Jackson, Mississippi

John Keith, MD
Assistant Professor of Emergency Medicine
University of Mississippi Medical Center
Jackson, Mississippi

Anna Lerant, MD
Associate Professor of Anesthesiology
University of Mississippi Medical Center
Jackson, Mississippi

Loretta Jackson Williams, MD, PhD
Associate Professor of Emergency Medicine
University of Mississippi Medical Center
Jackson, Mississippi

Christopher Decker
Fourth-year Medical Student
University of Mississippi School of Medicine
Jackson, Mississippi

Nathan Shefveland
Fourth-year Medical Student
University of Mississippi School of Medicine
Jackson, Mississippi

Preface

The idea for this book grew out of an institutional need for a relatively concise primer on the basics of pain management and procedural sedation. Experience at our institution has clearly demonstrated that current medical school curriculum and house-officer training provides little formal education in either pain management or procedural sedation. As such, practice may be variably effective and guided more often by habit than by fact. Often also missing is the ability to use a "balanced" approach to pain management, in which techniques and agents are combined, e.g., neural blockade and parenteral therapy.

This book is therefore intended to help fill this gap and provide a broad introduction to the basics of acute pain management and procedural sedation. Each chapter has been written to try to deliver the essential key concepts that might ideally be communicated at the bedside or on clinical rounds.

Our intent is to provide a concise yet formalized, organized pocket guide to pain management and procedural sedation. We envision this text to be applicable for any non-anesthesiologist who routinely provides procedural sedation or regularly writes for oral or parenteral analgesics. Our intent is to provide a quick "how to," along with basic pharmacology and considerations of alternative agents and methods, so that any practitioner has a more versatile approach to these techniques.

Our target audience is intended to be **primarily** medical students and non-anesthesiology house officers. We did include a chapter on epidural and intrathecal analgesia so that this book might also be of use to anesthesia personnel managing an acute pain service.

We acknowledge that many of the subjects covered are areas of pain management and sedation practices for which comparative data are rather scant; we have done our best to represent solid and accepted practice guidelines and to provide reasonable clinical advice based on our experience and that of colleagues.

We truly hope you find this useful and informative. We would very much appreciate feedback and/or suggestions on how to improve this book and make it more user-friendly. Please e-mail suggestions or observations to: wphillips@emergmed.umsmed.edu

William James Phillips, MD
John Keith, MD
Anna Lerant, MD
Loretta Jackson Williams, MD, PhD

Contents

Glossary and Acute Pain Measurements

John Keith

I. PAIN

Pain is defined by the International Association for the Study of Pain as "an unpleasant sensory and emotional experience associated with actual or potential tissue damage, or described in terms of such damage." Pain may be classified in several ways: acute or chronic, somatic, visceral, or neuropathic.

A. Acute pain

1. *Acute pain* or *inflammatory pain* usually results from tissue damage or noxious stimuli.
   a. When tissue damage occurs, pain receptors called *nociceptors* are activated by biochemical intermediaries of inflammation (leukotrienes, bradykinins, histamine, and other factors).
   b. Once activated, these receptors send impulses through the peripheral nerve, entering the spinal cord to synapse with higher order neurons.
   c. The impulse ascends in specific spinal tracts to cerebral centers for interpretation, thus producing the sensation of pain.
2. Acute pain usually results from an identifiable pathologic condition.
3. It serves an evolutionary role, warning an individual of potential injury or illness and preventing the worsening of an existing pathology.
4. It often involves activation of the sympathetic nervous system, producing increased heart rate (HR), blood pressure (BP), respiratory rate (RR), and symptoms of anxiety.

B. Chronic pain

1. *Chronic pain* or *neuropathic pain* is considered a distinct condition from acute pain.
2. Unlike acute pain, there is no evolutionary role for chronic pain.
3. Chronic pain is thought to result from central nervous system changes that alter the processing of stimuli, producing pain in the absence of inflammatory markers.
4. It is important to realize that many treatments for acute pain, including nonsteroidal anti-inflammatory drugs (NSAIDs) and opioids, may have little beneficial effect on chronic pain.
5. The spinal cord changes (*neuroplasticity*) that signal the transition from acute to chronic pain may begin very soon after injury.
   a. Many practitioners believe that inadequate treatment of acute pain syndromes may contribute to the development of a chronic pain state.
   b. Hence the caveat: **Treat acute pain aggressively and early!**

II. TYPES OF ACUTE PAIN

Acute pain is usually characterized as somatic, visceral, or neuropathic in origin.

A. Somatic pain

1. Somatic pain results from the triggering of nociceptors in the skin, musculoskeletal system, and body walls.
2. This pain is usually constant and well localized.
3. Causes of somatic pain include inflammation and micro or macro trauma.

B. Visceral pain

1. Pain felt from the viscera is usually perceived differently than somatic pain.
2. It is usually ill defined and may be poorly located. It also may be perceived in a site distal to the organ that is actually being damaged.
3. Visceral pain may result from four causes:
a. Ischemia
b. Inflammation with chemical stimulation
c. Overdistention of a hollow viscus
d. Spasm of a hollow viscus
4. Visceral pain is often associated with nausea and other systemic symptoms, whereas these symptoms are relatively rare in pure somatic pain.

C. Neuropathic pain

1. This pain typically originates from specific damage to a neural structure.
2. Examples include peripheral nerve injury (e.g., ischemic, crush), spinal cord injury, and herpes zoster.
3. The painful zone is typically in the dermatome of the damaged nerve but may rapidly spread to involve adjacent dermatomes.
4. Neuropathic pain is often an ill-defined burning, dysesthetic pain stimulated by modest provocation such as light touch or movement.
5. It may be accompanied by signs of autonomic hyperactivity in the painful zone, such as hyperemia or vasoconstriction and hyperhidrosis.

III. ACUTE PAIN ASSESSMENT

Pain is subjective and due to the interaction of many complex factors, both physiologic and psychological. **There are no objective tests or physical exam findings that reliably reproduce an individual's experience of pain.** It is important to assess pain and record an objective measurement of pain intensity to formulate a treatment plan.

A. Numerical rating scale

1. Individuals are asked to rate pain on a scale of 0 to 10, with 0 representing no pain and 10 representing the worst possible pain (Fig. 1-1).

No pain   0   1   2   3   4   5   6   7   8   9   10   Worst pain possible

Circle one number from 0 to 10

FIG. 1-1

Numerical pain scale. *(From Littman GS, Walker BR, Schneider BE: Reassessment of verbal and visual analog ratings in analgesic studies. Clin Pharmacol Ther 38(1):16–23, 1985.)*

2. Does not require written material and is sensitive in determining change in pain intensity in the acute setting

B. Visual analog scale
1. A 100-mm line, oriented horizontally and bounded at each end by verbal descriptors of pain intensity, from no pain at the left to worst possible pain at the right (Fig. 1-2)
2. Patients indicate with a mark their intensity of pain.
3. A change of 13 mm is indicative of a significant change in pain perception.
4. Reliable and reproducible measure of pain intensity
5. Requires the use of written materials

C. Faces pain scale
1. Developed for the assessment of pain in children or individuals with limited literacy
2. Composed of facial images; individuals are asked which facial image best matches his or her pain (Fig. 1-3).
3. Reliable and reproducible measurement of pain intensity

Least possible pain   Indicate the severity of your pain below   Most possible pain

Indicate by placing a single mark through the line at the appropriate point

FIG. 1-2

Visual analog scale. *(From Littman GS, Walker BR, Schneider BE: Reassessment of verbal and visual analog ratings in analgesic studies. Clin Pharmacol Ther 38(1):16–23, 1985.)*

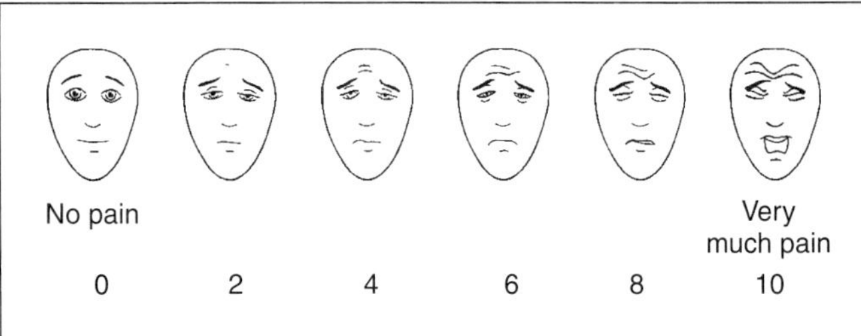

FIG. 1-3

Faces pain scale. In the instructions, say: *"These faces show how much something can hurt. This face [point to left-most face] shows no pain. The faces show more and more pain [point to each from left to right] up to this one [point to right-most face]—it shows very much pain. Point to the face that shows how much you hurt [right now]."* Score the chosen face 0, 2, 4, 6, 8, or 10, counting left to right, so 0 = no pain and 10 = very much pain. Do not use words like *happy* and *sad*. This scale is intended to measure how children feel inside, not how their faces look. *(From Hicks CL, von Baeyer CL, Spafford P, et al: The faces pain scale—revised: Toward a common metric in pediatric pain measurement. Pain 93:173–183, 2001. Used with permission from the International Association for the Study of Pain. This scale is available at* http://www.painsourcebook.ca.*)*

BIBLIOGRAPHY

Fink WA Jr. The pathophysiology of acute pain. *Emerg Med Clin North Am* 2005; 23(2):277–284.

Todd KH. Pain assessment instruments for use in the emergency department. *Emerg Med Clin North Am* 2005; 23(2):285–295.

Wah JA. Pain management in the hospitalized patient. *Med Clin North Am* 2002; 86:771–795.

Acute Pain Management

John Keith

I. OLIGOANALGESIA

A. Although patients often seek medical attention because of pain, physicians historically have focused first on identifying the etiology of the pain, with its alleviation being a secondary concern.

B. This problem was first identified in the late 1980s but still continues to be an issue, both in inpatient and outpatient settings. As an example, recent studies reveal that only 33% to 66% of patients who present to emergency departments in acute pain receive analgesics.

C. The current standard of care includes simultaneous treatment of pain while searching for the diagnosis of a patient's underlying condition!

II. OPIOIDS

A. Origin

1. Opium, a heterogeneous drug derived from milky exudate of the opium poppy, has been used to control human discomfort for more than 5000 years.
2. Morphine was first isolated in 1806, and other opium alkaloids, including papaverine and codeine, were soon isolated and began to replace unrefined opium in clinical practice.

B. Opioid receptors

1. Opioids exert their effects on receptors for endogenous human opioid peptides, including endorphins, enkephalins, and dynorphins found within the central nervous system (CNS), adrenal medulla, nerve plexus, gastric exocrine glands, and intestines.
2. These peptides have multiple roles, including the modulation of pain, neurohumoral transmission, and neurohormonal effects.
3. Three different types of opioid receptors are recognized: mu (μ), delta (δ), and kappa (κ).
a. μ Receptors mediate:
    (1) Supraspinal analgesia
    (2) Physical dependence
    (3) Euphoria
    (4) Sedation
    (5) Respiratory depression
    (6) Constipation

(7) Orthostatic hypotension
(8) Arteriolar and venous vessel dilation
b. δ Receptors mediate:
(1) Spinal analgesia
(2) Euphoria
(3) Potentate μ-receptor analgesia
c. κ Receptors mediate:
(1) Spinal analgesia
(2) Sedation
(3) Mitosis
(4) Supraspinal analgesia

C. Opioid types

1. Opioids may be either full or partial agonists, antagonists, or mixed agonist-antagonists.
2. Agonists occupy the opioid receptor and exert analgesic effect.
3. Partial agonists occupy the opioid receptor, resulting in a lesser degree of analgesia than a full agonist—hence the observed ceiling effect.
4. Antagonists bind to opioid receptors without eliciting analgesic effect. Antagonists can prevent opioid agonists from occupying opioid receptors. Clinically useful antagonists bind to the receptors rapidly and have a higher affinity for the receptors than agonists.
5. Mixed agonist-antagonists are agonists at κ receptors and block the μ receptors, hence the observed ceiling effect.

D. Opioid uses

1. Opioids are the most potent and effective analgesics available.
2. Pure opioid agonists exert their effects centrally (spinal cord, midbrain, and cortex) and produce dose-dependent analgesia without the "ceiling effect" of analgesics like nonsteroidal anti-inflammatory drugs (NSAIDs) and acetaminophen.
3. Can be used to treat diarrhea and gastrointestinal hypermotility by slowing of peristalsis
4. Lessen anxiety and excitation and induce a feeling of well-being
5. May be used in acute coronary syndromes and acute pulmonary edema to decrease sympathetic output and as venodilators

E. Routes of administration

1. Opioids can be administered by a number of routes, including PO, parenteral, rectal, sublingual, transdermal, transmucosal, intrathecal, and epidural.
2. Generally, the maximal analgesic effect occurs 60 to 90 minutes after oral dosing, 30 minutes after IM injection, and 2 to 6 minutes after IV injection.
3. Intrathecal onset relies on cerebrospinal fluid (CSF) migration to the painful spinal segment.
4. Epidural onset relies on volume spread in the epidural space and later diffusion across the dura to spinal roots.

F. Opioid dosing

1. There is a wide interindividual variation in the response to analgesics.
2. Because of the lack of a ceiling effect, the correct dose of opioids is the one that relieves the patient's pain.
3. The most effective means for providing adequate analgesia is to start with an initial weight-based dose and titrate upward with multiple small increases in dosage until adequate analgesia is achieved.
4. A recent study confirmed that morphine sulfate at a dose of 0.1 mg/kg is not adequate to relieve pain in most emergency department patients and that titration of additional doses is necessary for many patients.
5. Although any pure μ agonist would relieve severe pain if it could be tolerated in adequate doses, many have dose-limiting side effects that appear before adequate analgesia is achieved.
6. The choice of opioid for a specific patient should be individualized based on both the characteristics of the patient and the adverse effect profile of the drug (Fig. 2-1).

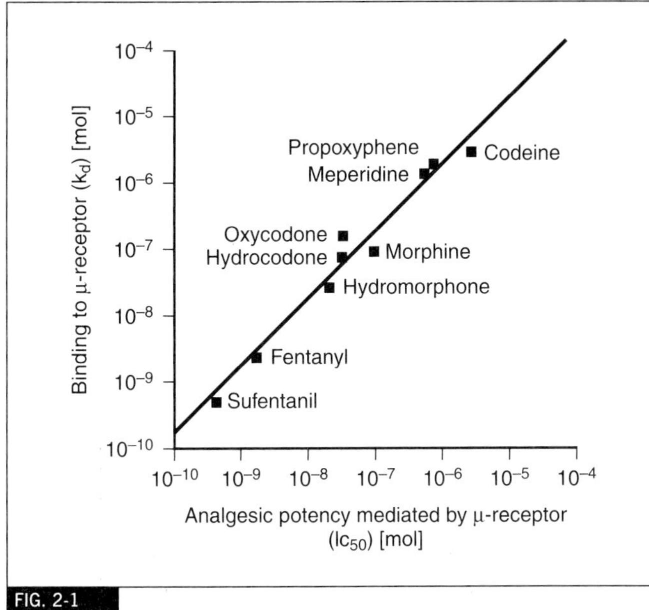

FIG. 2-1

Analgesic potency of opiate drugs correlates with μ-opiate receptor binding. *(Data from Creese I, Snyder SH: Receptor binding and pharmacological activity of opiates in the guinea-pig intestine. J Pharmacol Exp Ther 194:205–219, 1975.)*

G. Understanding lipid solubility

1. Opioids exert their analgesic and euphoric effects mainly on the CNS.
2. If an opioid is administered or absorbed into the vascular system, it must cross the blood-brain barrier to exert its effects.
3. The ability to cross the blood-brain barrier is known as the *diffusion potential* and is related to the lipid solubility of the drug.
4. The lipid diffusion index (LDI) is the ratio of the diffusion potential of an opioid compared with that of morphine.
5. Fentanyl has an LDI of 160, meperidine of 14.
6. As a general rule, the higher the LDI, the more likely it is to produce euphoria in excess of its analgesia.

III. INTRAVENOUS OPIOIDS

A. Overview of intravenous opioids

1. Morphine is the prototypic parenteral analgesic for the treatment of severe acute pain.
2. Because of its effectiveness, relative lack of toxicity, longer duration of action, and lesser euphoric tendency, morphine should be the opioid of first choice for the parenteral treatment of severe acute pain.
3. Other μ agonists such as hydromorphone, fentanyl, and meperidine are also used parentally but rarely offer advantages over morphine and often have disadvantages. These agents should be reserved for when morphine is contraindicated.
4. Less commonly used μ agonists include levorphanol, methadone, and oxymorphone, but there is limited experience with the use of these agents to treat acute pain in the ambulatory or inpatient setting.
5. Levorphanol (Levo-Dromoran) is the only commercially available agent of the morphinan series. The effects of this agent parallel those of morphine, with a potentially longer duration of action and less nausea and vomiting. The fact that this drug may also exhibit some κ agonist effects explains the incomplete cross-tolerance between this agent and morphine. Typical doses are 2 mg given PO or SC every 6 to 8 hours. It is not typically used intravenously.
6. Dextromethorphan is the D-isomer of levorphanol. It has minimal analgesic effects (possibly an *N*-methyl-D-aspartate [NMDA] antagonist) but elevates the central coughing threshold and is marketed as an antitussive agent.
7. Mixed opioid agonists-antagonists, including pentazocine, butorphanol, nalbuphine, and buprenorphine, are rarely indicated in acute pain. A ceiling effect limits their effectiveness in analgesia, and they may precipitate acute withdrawal in patients physically dependent on pure μ agonists.

B. Selected intravenous opioids

1. Morphine sulfate

a. Overview

    (1) Morphine is the prototypical opioid, first isolated from the opium poppy in 1806.

    (2) Its primary effects result from its interaction with μ receptors in the CNS.

    (3) Its primary therapeutic actions include analgesia and sedation.

    (4) Morphine sulfate is indicated for the relief of moderate to severe pain. It is also the narcotic agent of choice in the managing of pain associated with acute coronary syndrome (ACS) and the treatment of acutely decompensated congestive heart failure (CHF).

    (5) Morphine is the standard for making opioid conversions: The potencies of all other opioids are established relative to morphine.

b. Indications and usage

    (1) For moderate to severe pain in patients with no evidence of decreased intravascular volume, **the starting dose of morphine should be 0.1 mg/kg.**

    (2) **It may then be titrated upward in dosages of 2 to 4 mg every 5 to 10 minutes** until adequate analgesia is achieved.

    (3) The dose should be **reduced by 50%** in elderly patients, in the setting of renal failure, in patients with volume loss or hemorrhage, or in the setting of possible right ventricular infarction.

    (4) Onset of action is immediate for IV administration, 20 to 30 minutes for IM or SC administration, and about 1 hour for PO administration.

    (5) Duration of action is **2 to 3 hours.**

    (6) A recent study confirmed that morphine sulfate at a dose of 0.1 mg/kg may not be adequate to relieve pain in most emergency department patients and that titration of additional doses is necessary for many patients.

c. Metabolism

    (1) Morphine is metabolized in the liver with two active metabolites that require renal clearance.

    (2) These metabolites, **morphine 6-glucuronide (M6G) and morphine 3-glucuronide (M3G), may accumulate in elderly patients and in those with decreased renal function, producing enhanced opioid effects and CNS depression.**

d. Side effects

    (1) Like all opioids, morphine causes pruritus, nausea, constipation, and dizziness.

    (2) Compared with other opioids, morphine may cause more histamine release with resultant pruritus and rarely hypotension.

    (3) It is common to see localized urticaria tracking along forearm veins after IV morphine administration. This may be treated with antihistamines and **should not be considered an allergic reaction.**

    (4) Recent evidence places the incidence of increased biliary spasm to the level of a medical myth. **Morphine is NOT contraindicated in acute cholelithiasis or nephrolithiasis.**

e. Advantages

(1) Should be the drug of first choice when parenteral control of moderate to severe pain is indicated

(2) Produces less euphoria than more lipophilic opioids such as meperidine or hydromorphone

(3) Decreases myocardial workload and myocardial oxygen demand in the setting of cardiac ischemia

f. Disadvantages

(1) Dosing and schedule may need to be reduced in elderly patients and those with renal insufficiency.

(2) Strong histamine release may require co-administration of an antihistamine.

g. Clinical pearls

(1) IV morphine sulfate at a starting dose of 0.1–0.15 mg/kg should be the drug of first choice for the treatment of severe acute pain in healthy adult patients.

(2) The dose may then be titrated upward by 2- to 4-mg increments every 10 to 15 minutes until adequate analgesia can be achieved.

(3) The starting dose should be reduced by 50% in elderly patients, those with renal failure, patients with ACS, and those with possible volume depletion due to trauma.

2. Meperidine (Demerol)

a. Overview

(1) Meperidine HCl is a highly lipid-soluble synthetic narcotic analgesic structurally similar to **atropine,** with analgesic actions similar to those of morphine while maintaining many of its anticholinergic effects.

(2) The principal actions of therapeutic value are analgesia and sedation.

b. Indications and usage

(1) Meperidine is indicated for the relief of moderate to severe pain, for preoperative medication, for support of anesthesia, and for obstetric analgesia.

(2) Meperidine, in 60- to 80-mg parenteral doses, is about equivalent in analgesic effect to 10 mg of morphine.

(3) Standard parenteral dosing is 0.5 to 1.0 mg/kg IV, then titrated in 0.2- to 0.5-mg/kg increments every 5 to 10 minutes until complete analgesia is achieved or side effects predominate.

(4) The onset of action is slightly more rapid than with morphine, and the duration of action is slightly shorter (2 to 3 hours).

(5) It may be administered by the PO, IV, IM, or SC route.

c. Metabolism

(1) Ninety percent is converted in the liver by the cytochrome P-450 system to **normeperidine,** which is an active metabolite with decreased analgesic effects but increased neuroexcitatory effects, including anxiety, confusion, dysphoria, hallucinations, hyperreflexia, myoclonus, and occasional seizures.

- (2) Because of first-pass metabolism, normeperidine levels are higher in patients taking oral meperidine than in those on parenteral therapy.
- (3) Normeperidine has a longer half-life than meperidine, which can lead to its accumulation and increasing neurotoxicity, especially in elderly patients and patients with renal dysfunction.
- (4) Because normeperidine is not an opioid, its neurotoxic effects are not reversed by naloxone.
- d. Advantages: Meperidine has no clear clinical advantages in relation to other opioids other than potentially causing less constipation on a chronic basis. This may be due to its lipid solubility and ability to enter the CNS and produce analgesia at lower equianalgesic doses.
- e. Disadvantages
  - (1) An active metabolite (normeperidine) causes CNS excitation and possibly seizures, especially in elderly patients and those with diminished renal function.
  - (2) Meperidine is contraindicated in patients who are receiving monoamine oxidase (MAO) inhibitors and in those who have recently received such agents.
  - (3) It has a shorter duration of action than morphine.
  - (4) Significant increased euphoria and abuse potential compared with morphine or hydromorphone.
  - (5) Negative inotropic and positive chronotropic action.
  - (6) No more potent than 650 mg of acetaminophen when administered orally with increased abuse liability.
- f. Clinical pearl: Meperidine offers many disadvantages compared with morphine and no clinical advantages. It is therefore rarely the opioid of choice for the treatment of acute pain either orally or parenterally, including pain from biliary spasm.
3. Hydromorphone (Dilaudid)
a. Hydromorphone HCl is a moderately lipid-soluble hydrogenated ketone of morphine first synthesized in the early 20th century.
b. Indications and usage
  - (1) Hydromorphone HCl is indicated for the relief of moderate to severe pain.
  - (2) It is approved by the U.S. Food and Drug Administration (FDA) **ONLY** in patients who are narcotic tolerant, but is often used in narcotic-naïve patients in the clinical setting.
  - (3) Hydromorphone in a dose of 1.5 mg produces analgesia equal to that produced by 10 mg of morphine (typical conversion with morphine = 1:7).
  - (4) Usual starting parenteral dose is 1 to 2 mg (.01 to .02 mg/kg) IV administered over 2 to 3 minutes and titrated to effect.
  - (5) Less first-pass effect than morphine, so PO to IV dosing conversion is 2:1, compared with 3:1 for morphine.

    (6) Administered by IV route, it has an immediate onset, whereas it has a slightly more rapid onset than morphine when given by the IM or SC owing to its increased lipid solubility.

    (7) The duration of action of hydromorphone is usually 2 to 3 hours, although it may be up to 4 to 5 hours in narcotic-naïve patients.

c. Metabolism: Hydromorphone is dehydrogenated in the liver to morphine. It has no other active metabolites.

d. Advantages

    (1) Hydromorphone has a rapid onset of action and small dose for IM or SC administration.

    (2) Hydromorphone tends to produce less euphoria than meperidine, although more than morphine.

    (3) Elderly patients and those who have renal impairment tend to tolerate sustained-release oral hydromorphone better than sustained-release oral morphine with less drowsiness and cognitive impairment.

e. Disadvantages

    (1) Shorter duration of action than morphine

    (2) More euphoria than morphine

f. Clinical pearls

    (1) Hydromorphone might be used preferentially over morphine in **elderly patients and those with renal impairment.**

    (2) Hydromorphone might be used preferentially over morphine in patients receiving **IM or SC opioids** because of its more rapid absorption and decreased volume of injection.

    (3) **Although chemically similar, this is an excellent substitute for patients with a true morphine allergy.**

4. Fentanyl (Sublimaze)

a. Overview

    (1) Fentanyl citrate is a potent, highly lipid-soluble synthetic opioid of the phenylpiperidine group.

    (2) Useful for short-term analgesia and sedation, most commonly in the perioperative setting or during procedural sedation

b. Indications and usage

    (1) Because of its lipid solubility, fentanyl has a rapid onset of action of 3 to 5 minutes and a **duration of analgesic action of 30 minutes.** It is then redistributed from the CNS into tissues with an elimination half-life of 3 hours.

    (2) A dose of 100 μg (0.1 mg; 2.0 mL) is about equivalent in analgesic activity to 10 mg of morphine or 75 mg of meperidine (morphine-to-fentanyl conversion = 100:1).

    (3) Starting dose of fentanyl for acute pain should be **1 to 2 μg/kg,** then titrated every 3 to 5 minutes in **0.25- to 0.5-μg/kg** increments until pain is relieved or side effects predominate. (Analgesia is equated with sympatholysis, seen at 0.5 μg/kg).

    (4) Transdermal patches **(Duragesic)** are available for long-acting analgesia in patients with chronic pain. These patches have a

very slow onset of action, requiring about a day to reach steady state, and are **rarely appropriate** for use in acute pain syndromes.

(5) Lollipops and orally dissolving tablets are available. Extreme caution should be used because high blood levels are attained rapidly. The primary application for these preparations is when IV access is unavailable in the significantly opioid-tolerant patient.

c. Metabolism: Primarily transformed in the liver to inactive metabolites

d. Advantages

(1) Rapid onset of action compared with morphine

(2) Short half-life

(3) Produces **less histamine release** than morphine-like opioids and thus has fewer cardiovascular effects and less hypotension

(4) Less emetic activity than morphine or meperidine

e. Disadvantages

(1) Short duration of action, may require more frequent dosing

(2) Respiratory depression may last longer than analgesia.

f. Clinical pearls

(1) Fentanyl might be preferentially used over morphine for the relief of pain in patients who may be **volume depleted or are dependent on cardiac preload.**

(2) Exhibits excellent hemodynamic stability!

(3) Also available as an Oralet/lollipop (Actiq), which shows extremely rapid systemic uptake, as does the buccal dissolving capsule.

IV. ORAL OPIOIDS

A. Overview of oral opioids

1. Oral opioids are often combined with other analgesics such as acetaminophen, ibuprofen, or aspirin to provide a synergistic increase in efficacy in treating acute pain.

2. Oxycodone and hydrocodone are commonly used μ agonists for the treatment of moderate to severe acute pain.

3. Oral morphine, meperidine, and hydromorphone are also used in the treatment of acute pain, although they are used less frequently in this setting than either hydrocodone or oxycodone.

4. Historically, propoxyphene and codeine have been used frequently for acute pain. Recent literature calls into question their roles as first-line medications for the treatment of acute pain due to their relative ineffectiveness and side-effect profiles.

5. Methadone, levorphanol, and dihydrocodeine are rarely used in the treatment of acute pain.

6. Sustained-release preparations of morphine and oxycodone have been created. These preparations are valuable in the management of chronic pain; however, because of their delayed onset of action and possibility of redosing, they should not be used for acute pain control in non-opioid-tolerant patients.

7. Exceptions include cases in which pain is immediately controlled with parenterally titrated agents while simultaneously administering a longer-acting oral agent to provide longer duration coverage.

B. Selected oral opioids

1. Hydrocodone

a. Overview

   (1) Hydrocodone is a semi-synthetic opioid analgesic and antitussive.

   (2) Hydrocodone is generally considered to be the most potent Schedule III or lower opioid.

   (3) Hydrocodone is a prodrug; it is metabolized to hydromorphone in the liver.

b. Indication and usage

   (1) Hydrocodone is indicated for the oral treatment of **moderate to severe pain.**

   (2) For acute pain, multiple combination products exist either with acetaminophen (e.g., Vicodin, Lorcet) or with ibuprofen (e.g., Vicoprofen) in doses of 2.5 to 20 mg, with a usual starting dose of **5 to 10 mg of hydrocodone every 4 to 6 hours.**

   (3) Hydrocodone-acetaminophen preparation dosing is limited by acetaminophen content, and care should be used to ensure the **total daily acetaminophen dosage does not exceed 4 g/day.**

   (4) A recent clinical trial demonstrated analgesic effects similar to oxycodone at 30 and 60 minutes in patients with acute fractures.

   (5) There was no significant difference in the incidence of nausea and vomiting between the two drugs, although hydrocodone was associated with increased constipation.

c. Advantages

   (1) Superior analgesia with fewer gastrointestinal (GI) effects compared with codeine or propoxyphene

   (2) Classified as Schedule III by the FDA as opposed to Schedule II for oxycodone

   (3) Similar analgesic effects to oxycodone

d. Disadvantages

   (1) May be more constipating than oxycodone

   (2) May have a greater abuse liability than codeine

e. Clinical pearls

   (1) Hydrocodone is the most potent and effective Schedule III opioid analgesic available (Schedule III as a combination agent, Lortab; Schedule II as a sole agent) and should be considered the oral opioid of choice for the oral treatment of moderate to severe acute pain.

   (2) Hydrocodone-acetaminophen combinations (e.g., Lortab, Vicodin) with 5 mg of hydrocodone should be prescribed for moderate pain in most individuals. Dosing is 1 to 2 tablets every 4 to 6 hours.

    (3) Hydrocodone-acetaminophen combinations (e.g., Lortab, Vicodin) with 10 mg of hydrocodone should be prescribed for severe pain in most individuals. Dosing is 1 to 2 tablets every 4 to 6 hours.

    (4) Hydrocodone-ibuprofen combinations (Vicoprofen) may be considered as an alternative for moderate to severe pain if a patient has no contraindications to NSAID use.

2. Oxycodone

a. Overview

    (1) Oxycodone is a semi-synthetic pure opioid agonist with a mechanism of action similar to codeine.

    (2) In the setting of acute pain, oxycodone exhibits a synergistic effect with acetaminophen or ibuprofen.

    (3) It is an effective analgesic offering superior analgesia to codeine with fewer GI side effects.

    (4) Oxycodone is classified as a **Schedule II** drug by the Drug Enforcement Agency (DEA) and in many states requires specialized prescribing documentation.

    (5) Oxycodone may exhibit greater euphoria than codeine, and this, coupled with its favorable side-effect profile, may lead to a **greater abuse potential.**

    (6) A recent clinical trial demonstrated analgesic effects similar to hydrocodone at 30 and 60 minutes in patients with acute fractures. There was no significant difference in the incidence of nausea and vomiting between the two drugs, although hydrocodone was associated with increased constipation.

b. Indication and usage

    (1) Oxycodone is indicated for the relief of moderate to severe pain.

    (2) The usual adult starting dose of oxycodone is 5 to 20 mg PO every 4 to 6 hours.

    (3) Because of its synergistic effects with ibuprofen and acetaminophen, it is usually administered as a combination product with acetaminophen (e.g., Tylox, Percocet) for acute pain.

    (4) These products generally contain between 2.5 and 10 mg of oxycodone with varying strengths of acetaminophen.

    (5) Oxycodone-acetaminophen preparation dosing is limited by acetaminophen content, and care should be used to ensure the total daily acetaminophen dosage does not exceed 4 g/day.

    (6) Both immediate-release and sustained-release preparations are available without acetaminophen; however, these preparations have been shown to be inferior to the combination products in the setting of acute pain.

    (7) OxyContin is a sustained-release form of oxycodone that is usually administered on a twice-daily basis. Because of its delayed onset of action and problems with dependency, misuse, and diversion, this formulation should rarely be used as a first-line treatment for acute pain.

c. Adverse effects
  (1) Side effects include nausea, headache, dizziness, and drowsiness. These side effects are dose related and rarely severe.
  (2) At 5 mg, oxycodone has a similar rate of adverse effects as placebo; however, increasing doses result in significantly more side effects.
d. Advantages
  (1) It is an effective analgesic offering superior analgesia to codeine with fewer GI side effects.
  (2) It may be less constipating than hydrocodone.
e. Disadvantages
  (1) Oxycodone is classified as a **Schedule II** drug by the DEA and in many states requires specialized prescribing documentation.
  (2) Oxycodone may exhibit greater euphoria than codeine, and this, coupled with its favorable side-effect profile, may lead to a **greater abuse potential.**
  (3) Sustained-release oxycodone (OxyContin) is strongly associated with dependency, misuse, and diversion.
f. Clinical pearls
  (1) Oxycodone-acetaminophen combinations in dosages of 5 to 20 mg of oxycodone every 4 to 6 hours should be considered a second-line oral opioid for the treatment of moderate to severe pain.
  (2) Sustained-release (OxyContin) and immediate-release oxycodone (OxyIR) products not containing acetaminophen are inferior to combination products in the setting of acute pain and should be used with caution in acute pain due to problems with dependency, misuse, and diversion.
3. Codeine
a. Overview
  (1) Codeine is a methylated alkaloid of opium first isolated in the early 1800s.
  (2) It is absorbed more completely than morphine and **is metabolized by hepatic enzymes to morphine** and other active metabolites.
  (3) Historically, codeine has been the most commonly prescribed opioid. Codeine has usually been given in combination with acetaminophen for analgesia.
  (4) It is a moderately effective analgesic for mild to moderate pain, but GI side effects often prevent toleration of dose escalation above 60 mg.
b. Indications and dosing
  (1) Codeine is indicated for the treatment of mild to moderate pain
  (2) The usual adult dose is 30 to 60 mg of codeine combined with acetaminophen every 4 to 6 hours. Codeine dosage is limited by GI side effects and the acetaminophen content of combination products.
  (3) Increasing codeine dosage above 60 mg produces relatively less analgesia when compared with the increase in nausea, constipation, and sedation patients experience.

c. Side effects
  (1) Side effects are dose related and include pruritus, nausea, constipation, sedation, and dizziness.
  (2) Ten percent of the population has a genetically limited ability to metabolize codeine into morphine. These individuals experience codeine's adverse effects without obtaining analgesia.
d. Advantage: Because of its large incidence of GI complications at doses that have limited euphoric effects, codeine is abused less frequently than hydrocodone or oxycodone.
e. Disadvantage: Patients receiving codeine experience significantly less analgesia and significantly more side effects when compared with hydrocodone or oxycodone.
f. Clinical pearls
  (1) Because of its relatively weak analgesic properties and significant side effects, codeine **should not be considered a first-line medication for the treatment of acute pain.**
  (2) If this agent were not converted to morphine, it would likely be nothing more than an antitussive.
  (3) If codeine is administered to a patient, **the dose should not exceed 60 mg** every 4 hours, and **co-administration of a laxative** is recommended.
4. Propoxyphene
a. Overview
  (1) Propoxyphene is a low-potency opioid analgesic that was once one of the most prescribed agents for acute pain.
  (2) It is a relatively poor analgesic agent; studies show that it is only marginally if at all better than placebo.
  (3) Overdoses with this opioid can be toxic, with refractory seizures and respiratory depression leading to death. For these reasons, the use of propoxyphene compounds is decreasing.
b. Indication and dosage
  (1) Propoxyphene is only indicated for the treatment of mild to moderate pain. It is not indicated in the treatment of severe pain.
  (2) The usual dosage is 65 mg propoxyphene every 4 hours as needed for pain. The maximum recommended of propoxyphene is 390 mg/day.
  (3) A recent meta-analysis compared the combination of propoxyphene and acetaminophen with acetaminophen alone. The propoxyphene combination demonstrated little analgesic effect over acetaminophen alone.
c. Metabolism
  (1) Like meperidine, propoxyphene is converted to an active metabolite norpropoxyphene.
  (2) This metabolite is a CNS stimulant as well as causing cardiac toxicity.
d. Side effects
  (1) Propoxyphene is associated with GI side effects similar to codeine.

(2) Taken in overdose, propoxyphene may cause seizures and cardiac conduction abnormalities.

e. Advantages and disadvantages

(1) Propoxyphene offers no significant advantages over other oral opioids.

(2) Propoxyphene is a weak analgesic, only indicated for mild to moderate pain, and has a side-effect profile out of proportion to its clinical efficacy.

(3) Propoxyphene is a dangerous drug in overdose with CNS and cardiac toxicity as well as the usual opioid toxidrome.

f. Clinical pearl: Because of its relatively weak analgesic properties (only marginally better than codeine) and its significant associated adverse effects both in routine use and overdose, **propoxyphene is not recommended for routine use for acute pain.**

V. NONOPIOID ORAL ANALGESICS AND NONSTEROIDAL ANTI-INFLAMMATORY DRUGS (NSAIDS)

A. Nonopioid oral analgesics

1. Acetaminophen

a. Overview

(1) Acetaminophen is a nonopioid analgesic and antipyretic without anti-inflammatory properties.

(2) The mechanism of analgesic action of acetaminophen remains unclear; its antipyretic effects are through actions on the hypothalamic heat-regulating center.

(3) Acetaminophen is an equally effective analgesic as aspirin with an improved safety profile.

(4) Acetaminophen in 1000-mg doses is as effective as NSAIDs in some acute pain indications like tension headache, but less effective in dental and menstrual pain.

(5) Acetaminophen should be considered a drug of choice for the initial management of osteoarthritis and for the treatment of fever in both children and adults.

(6) Acetaminophen is available over the counter as tablets, caplets, and liquid suspensions as well as suppositories.

(7) Acetaminophen is also available in a number of combination products both over the counter and by prescription.

(8) One problem is, given the ubiquitous nature of acetaminophen-containing products, care must be taken not to accidentally exceed the daily maximal dose.

b. Pharmacology

(1) Onset

(a) Acetaminophen is rapidly absorbed after oral or rectal administration, with peak levels of uncoated tablets occurring at 30 to 60 minutes.

(b) Extended-release acetaminophen preparations have a peak level occurring about 4 hours after ingestion.

(2) Half-life: The half-life of acetaminophen is 1 to 4 hours after absorption.

(3) Duration of action

    (a) 4 hours with oral administration of uncoated tablets

    (b) 8 hours with extended release preparations

(4) Metabolism and elimination: Acetaminophen is primarily metabolized in the liver, with more than 90% converted to glucuronide and sulfate conjugates and 5% excreted unchanged in the liver.

c. Indication and dosing

  (1) Acetaminophen is indicated for the treatment of mild to moderate pain and fever in adults and children.

  (2) Adult dosing: 650 to 1000 mg (1000 mg more efficacious) orally every 4 hours up to 4 times a day.

  (3) Pediatric dosing: 15 mg/kg every 4 to 6 hours up to 4 times a day.

d. Adverse effects

  (1) Common

    (a) Dermatologic: rash

    (b) Endocrine metabolic: hypothermia

  (2) Serious

    (a) Gastrointestinal: GI hemorrhage

    (b) Hepatic: hepatotoxicity

    (c) Renal: nephrotoxicity

    (d) Respiratory: pneumonitis

e. Advantages

  (1) Widely available safe analgesic and antipyretic available in multiple formulations and combination products.

  (2) Taken as directed, acetaminophen still has the best safety profile of any agent for the treatment of acute pain.

f. Disadvantages

  (1) No anti-inflammatory properties.

  (2) May be less efficacious than ibuprofen in conditions like dysmenorrhea and acute sprains and strains, for which peripheral antiprostaglandin effects are beneficial.

g. Clinical pearls

  (1) Acetaminophen in doses of **1000 mg** every 6 hours for adult patients or **15 mg/kg** in pediatric patients should be considered as a first-line medication for analgesia for mild to moderate pain.

  (2) Taken as directed, acetaminophen still has the **best safety profile of any agent for the treatment of acute pain.**

  (3) Caution should be taken **not to exceed a total daily dose of 4000 mg/day** of acetaminophen, especially if patients are using combination narcotic products or over-the-counter preparations containing acetaminophen.

2. Aspirin

a. Aspirin has not proved more effective than equal doses of acetaminophen or ibuprofen in acute pain. It has a worse safety profile

than acetaminophen and ibuprofen and therefore **is not recommended** as a first-line agent in acute pain.
b. Aspirin should be avoided in children with febrile illnesses because of its association with Reye's syndrome, a potentially fatal condition characterized by acute encephalopathy and fatty degeneration of the liver.
3. Tramadol (Ultram)
a. Overview
   (1) Tramadol is a central analgesic that produces its analgesic effect both by binding of both the parent drug and its M1 metabolite to μ opioid receptors and by weak inhibition of the uptake of norepinephrine and serotonin.
   (2) Tramadol in standard dosages appears to be a more effective analgesic than acetaminophen but less effective than opioids like hydrocodone and oxycodone.
   (3) It is available as a combination product with acetaminophen (**Ultracet** with 37.5 tramadol and 325 mg acetaminophen) that in limited studies appears to be more efficacious than acetaminophen with codeine but less efficacious than combinations products with hydrocodone or oxycodone.
   (4) It is also available as a sustained-release preparation for before-bedtime use.
   (5) Tramadol is not controlled under the Controlled Substances Act and has been promoted as having decreased abuse potential compared with more traditional opioids, although abuse and withdrawal symptoms have been reported.
   (6) It is used parenterally in Europe.
b. Pharmacology
   (1) Onset: Tramadol is rapidly absorbed after oral administration, with peak concentration of tramadol occurring at 2 hours and M1 at 3 hours.
   (2) Metabolism: Tramadol is metabolized in the liver to its active metabolite M1 and other metabolites that are eliminated in the urine.
   (3) Half-life: The plasma half-life of tramadol is 6 hours following a single dose and increases to 7 hours with repeated administration.
c. Indications and dosing
   (1) Tramadol is indicated for the treatment of moderate to severe pain in adult patients.
   (2) In adults, the dosage for acute pain is **50 to 100 mg** PO every **4 to 6 hours** not to exceed **400 mg a day.**
   (3) In patients with **creatinine clearance less than 30 mL/minute,** the dosing interval should be increased to every **12 hours,** and the dose should not exceed **200 mg/day.**
   (4) In patients with **cirrhosis,** the recommended adult dose is **50 mg** every **12 hours.**
   (5) In elderly patients, the dose should begin at the low end of the dosing range **(25 mg)** and slowly be titrated upward. In patient older than **75 years,** the dose should not exceed **300 mg per day.**

(6) **Tramadol-acetaminophen** (37.5/325) tablets are dosed **2 tablets every 4 to 6 hours for pain** not to exceed **8 tablets per day.**

d. Adverse effects

(1) Tramadol has a high incidence of CNS effects, including dizziness, headache, somnolence, and CNS stimulation.

(2) Tramadol also has a high incidence of nausea and vomiting, constipation, and dyspepsia.

(3) Serious neurotoxicity can occur in overdose, including seizure, agitation, coma, and respiratory depression.

e. Advantages

(1) May be more efficacious than acetaminophen or codeine.

(2) Is not a controlled substance under the Controlled Substances Act and might have a lower abuse liability than opioids such as hydrocodone or oxycodone.

f. Disadvantages

(1) Frequent adverse effects.

(2) Inferior efficacy to opioids like hydrocodone or oxycodone.

(3) Increased abuse liability compared with acetaminophen or NSAIDs.

g. Clinical pearls

(1) Because of its relative inferior efficacy compared with traditional opioids and its side-effect profile, tramadol might **not** be considered a first-line "solo" medication for the treatment of acute pain.

(2) It is an unusual analgesic with both a mild μ agonist effect and a tricyclic antidepressant (norepinephrine and serotonin reuptake blocker) effect. It is a chemical cousin of codeine.

(3) Its best use may be as a co-analgesic in combination with NSAIDS.

4. NSAIDs

a. NSAIDs may be used preferentially over acetaminophen in patients with tension headache, acute sprains or strains, and dysmenorrhea.

b. NSAIDs should be **used with caution** in patients with preexisting **history of peptic ulcer disease or upper GI bleed, chronic renal insufficiency, or congestive heart failure or in patients taking angiotensin-converting enzyme (ACE) inhibitors, diuretics, glucocorticoids, oral anticoagulants, lithium, methotrexate, or phenytoin.**

c. NSAIDs have been shown to decrease experimental fracture healing and for this reason are **not recommended** for ongoing analgesia in patients during periods of **bone healing.**

B. NSAIDs

1. Overview

a. Salicylate-containing compounds, including willow bark, have been used for the treatment of acute pain and inflammation in Western medicine since the days of Ancient Greece.

b. Aspirin was introduced to medicine in 1899, whereas indomethacin and other agents were introduced in the 1940s and 1950s.

c. Nonsteroidal antiinflammatory drugs (NSAIDs) are a commonly prescribed group of analgesics and antipyretics that share a common mechanism of action of reversibly inhibiting the action of cyclooxygenase (COX).

d. The first agents specific for COX-2, celecoxib and rofecoxib, were introduced in 1999.

2. NSAID indications

a. NSAIDs are effective analgesics for mild to moderate pain. They have a low abuse potential and do not produce sedation or constipation. In the short term, NSAIDs may have a more favorable safety profile than opioids.

b. NSAIDs are superior to acetaminophen for musculoskeletal pain and may provide equivalent analgesia to the usual starting narcotics in renal colic and other painful pathologic conditions.

c. NSAIDs are commonly used for the treatment of acute painful conditions, including musculoskeletal sprains and strains, acute gouty flares, menstrual cramps, headaches, renal colic, and nonspecific pain and fever.

d. NSAIDS are also used in the chronic management of degenerative joint disease and inflammatory arthritis, usually at a higher dose than is necessary for the treatment of acute pain.

e. NSAIDs are equally effective antipyretics as acetaminophen and aspirin.

f. Although no individual NSAID has been shown to be superior in population-based studies, certain patients tend to respond better to individual drugs.

3. Physiology of COX

a. The COX enzymes are the first committed step in the synthesis of prostaglandins from arachidonic acid

b. COX exists in two distinct forms; COX-1 and COX-2.

c. COX-1

    (1) COX-1 is expressed in all cells (constitutive) and involved in the regulation of homeostatic functions.

    (2) Its expression is not altered by inflammatory stimuli.

    (3) It is the dominant isoform in mature platelets and the gastrointestinal mucosa.

d. COX-2

    (1) COX-2 has inducible expression when inflammatory cytokines, microbial products, or mitogens are present.

    (2) Independent of its role in inflammation, COX-2 also plays an important role in normal reproductive, renal, cardiovascular, and skeletal physiology.

e. Cardiovascular effects

    (1) COX-1 generates platelet thromboxane A_2, which has prothrombotic and vasoconstrictive effects. It is through the blockage of thromboxane A_2 that aspirin exerts its cardioprotective effects.

    (2) COX-1 and COX-2 both generate endothelial prostacyclin, which has vasodilatory and antiplatelet effects. Drugs that block production of

prostacyclin in excess of thromboxane such as COX-2 inhibitors may have prothrombotic effects and increase the risk for cardiovascular events.

4. Pharmacology of NSAIDs

a. NSAIDs inhibit the production of prostaglandins by competing with arachidonic acid for binding in the COX catalytic site.

b. Most traditional NSAIDs inhibit COX-1 and COX-2 to a similar extent.

c. COX-2-specific NSAIDs that have been introduced since 1999 predominately inhibit COX-2.

d. Most NSAIDs are completely absorbed from the GI tract following oral administration.

e. After absorption, most NSAIDs undergo significant protein binding. This protein binding can cause the displacement of other highly protein-bound drugs, particularly phenytoin and warfarin.

f. NSAIDs usually undergo hepatic metabolism, producing inactive metabolites that are excreted in the bile and urine.

g. Most NSAIDs are metabolized through the microsomal cytochrome P-450–containing mixed-function oxidase system.

h. Some of the variability of response to NSAIDs in individual patients is thought to be due to differing pharmacodynamic profiles.

5. NSAIDs in acute pain

a. The dose of NSAIDs sufficient to relieve acute pain is usually substantially lower than that necessary to produce anti-inflammatory effects.

b. The analgesic action of NSAIDs is likely to be due to inhibition of prostaglandin production both peripherally and centrally.

c. Unlike opioids, NSAIDs have a ceiling dose above which no additional analgesia is obtained.

d. Comparisons of NSAIDs usually demonstrate equivalent efficacy in patient populations, and there is no evidence that one NSAID is superior for a given indication (e.g., indomethacin for gout).

e. Certain patients may respond more favorably to individual NSAIDs. This is often relevant in patients who are undergoing long-term treatment with NSAIDs for chronic inflammatory conditions or degenerative arthritis.

f. Owing to the lack of large clinical trials demonstrating superiority of individual NSAIDs, the choice of an agent for acute pain should be based on cost and clinical familiarity.

g. Ibuprofen in starting dosages of 400 mg every 6 to 8 hours should be the first-line NSAID in the treatment of acute pain.

6. Adverse effects of NSAIDS

a. The primary adverse effects of NSAIDs that are not specific for COX-2 are on the gastrointestinal, renal, and platelet systems.

b. **Gastrointestinal effects**

(1) COX-1 inhibition of prostaglandin synthesis in the gastric mucosa is the central pathologic mechanism in adverse gastrointestinal effects in patients taking NSAIDs.

(2) Nonulcerative dyspepsia is the most common side effect associated with NSAID administration, affecting 10% to 20% of patients taking NSAIDs.

(3) The most serious side effect of NSAID use is the development of acute complications of NSAID-induced gastric ulcers, including life-threatening GI hemorrhage, perforation, or obstruction.

(4) The use of NSAIDs that are not specific for COX-2 is associated with a four-fold increase in the incidence of these complications, and the 1-year likelihood of ulcer-related hospitalization or death has been estimated to be 1% in NSAID users.

(5) Few data exist on the risk for short-term administration of NSAIDs for acute pain in patients with or without a history of peptic ulcer disease.

(6) COX-2–specific agents have been shown to be associated with a 50% relative risk reduction of clinically significant GI events and to be of the greatest benefit in the patients who are at highest risk for GI complications.

(7) In addition to the use of COX-2–specific agents, the risk for GI side effects may be reduced through the co-administration of proton pump inhibitors or misoprostol, whereas the beneficial effects of histamine-2 blockers are less clear, but because of a relatively high number needed to treat for effect demonstration, these measures should be reserved for high-risk patients.

c. Renal effects

(1) Vasodilatory prostaglandins produced by COX are important in maintaining renal blood flow.

(2) NSAIDs may cause increased sodium and water retention by blocking natriuresis in the ascending loop and the collecting system.

(3) In patients who are dehydrated, in CHF, or taking ACE inhibitors or diuretics, administration of an NSAID may result in renal ischemia and resultant acute renal insufficiency or acute renal failure.

(4) The risk for nephrotoxicity is dose dependent and most likely to occur during the first month of therapy.

(5) NSAID-mediated sodium retention may result in hypertension or worsening control of CHF.

(6) Hyperkalemia has been reported.

d. **Platelet effects:** Exhibited for the life of the platelet after aspirin use but shorter term and less profound with other NSAIDs.

e. **Cardiovascular effects:** Traditional NSAIDs antagonize the effect of both thromboxane (vasoconstrictive effect) and prostacyclin (vasodilatory effect). COX-2 inhibitors likely leave the former relatively unaffected, resulting in a predominant vasoconstrictive effect in the microcirculation.

f. **Hepatic effects**

(1) Small asymptomatic elevation in liver tests are relatively common in patients taking NSAIDs, whereas aspartate transaminase (AST) and alanine aminotransferase (ALT) elevation of 3 times or more the upper limit of normal have been reported in about 1% of patients.

(2) More severe hepatic reactions, including fulminant liver failure, have been reported in a small number of patients taking NSAIDs.

g. **Aspirin sensitive asthma:** In 10% to 20% of the general asthmatic population, ingestion of aspirin or of non-COX-2–specific NSAIDs may result in a severe exacerbation with naso-ocular reactions. This reaction is more common in patients with the triad of asthma, nasal polyposis, and vasomotor rhinitis.

h. **Bone healing**
   (1) Induction of COX-2 is important in regulation of bone formation and remodeling.
   (2) NSAIDs have been shown to decrease experimental fracture healing and for this reason are **not recommended** for ongoing analgesia in patients during periods of **bone healing.**

i. Drug interactions
   (1) NSAIDs have multiple drug interactions and should be used with caution in patients with preexisting history of peptic ulcer disease or upper GI bleed, chronic renal insufficiency, of CHF or patients taking ACE inhibitors, diuretics, glucocorticoids, oral anticoagulants, lithium, methotrexate, or phenytoin.
   (2) Use with great caution in elderly patients!
   (3) Oral anticoagulants: NSAIDs are protein bound and as such can displace bound warfarin; coupled with their antiplatelet effects, this can result in increased bleeding.
   (4) Phenytoin: NSAIDs can alter the hepatic metabolism and protein binding of phenytoin and may necessitate more frequent monitoring of phenytoin levels.
   (5) Glucocorticoids: Concurrent use of NSAIDs and glucocorticoids may increase the risk for peptic ulcer disease by significantly affecting prostaglandin synthesis in the gastric mucosa. When used in combination with glucocorticoids, NSAIDs should be used at the lowest dose possible and for the shortest feasible duration.
   (6) Antihypertensive agents: By decreasing natriuresis in the distal portion of the ascending loop and collecting system, NSAIDs may decrease the antihypertensive effects of ACE inhibitors, thiazide diuretics, and β blockers.
   (7) Diuretics
       (a) NSAID-induced reduction in renal blood flow may result in an increased risk for acute renal failure in patients taking diuretics.
       (b) Because the effects of NSAIDs are in the thick ascending loop, the diuretic and natriuretic properties of thiazides are unaffected, but the loop diuretics are adversely affected.
   (8) **Lithium:** By inhibiting natriuresis in the distal nephron, NSAIDs enhance the reabsorption of lithium and may cause an increase in lithium levels.

(9) **Methotrexate:** NSAIDs have been shown to alter the metabolism and decrease the clearance of methotrexate when concurrently administered and have been associated with severe toxicity.

7. COX-2 inhibitors

a. First introduced in 1999, COX-2 inhibitors represented a new class of NSAIDs specifically developed to have less effect on gastric prostaglandin E_2 production and a more favorable GI safety profile.

b. Celecoxib (Celebrex) was the first agent and was approved for use in osteoarthritis and rheumatoid arthritis but not for acute pain.

c. Rofecoxib (Vioxx) and valdecoxib (Bextra) were subsequently introduced and approved for acute pain application, including headache and dysmenorrhea.

d. COX-2 inhibitors were shown to have a 50% relative risk reduction for life-threatening GI complications compared with traditional NSAIDs and were widely marketed as a superior alternative to traditional NSAIDs.

e. There were no trials demonstrating superior efficacy of COX-2 agents over traditional NSAIDs, and the cost of treatment with COX-2 agents was typically 3 to 4 times as expensive.

f. Further studies revealed that rofecoxib (Vioxx) was associated with an almost four-fold increase in the incidence of serious thromboembolic events when compared with placebo.

g. The FDA requested the voluntary withdrawal of rofecoxib and valdecoxib from the U.S. market.

h. Celecoxib is the only COX-2 inhibitor currently approved for usage in the United States.

i. COX-2 inhibitors are no more efficacious in the treatment of acute pain than traditional NSAIDs and have not been shown to have an improved safety profile in short-term use. They are significantly more expensive than ibuprofen or naproxen without increased analgesic efficacy. They may be associated with increased risk for cardiovascular events and, given their lack of advantages in the acute setting, are not recommended for the treatment of acute pain.

C. Selected NSAIDs

1. Ibuprofen

a. Overview

(1) The most commonly used NSAID, ibuprofen is a propionic acid derivative with analgesic, anti-inflammatory, and antipyretic properties.

(2) Available in the United States over the counter as 200-mg tablets and as a liquid suspension containing 100 mg per 5 mL or 40 mg per 1 mL and by prescription in 300 mg, 400 mg, 600 mg, and 800 mg tablets.

(3) Ibuprofen has been shown to be as effective as aspirin in treating the pain and inflammation associated with rheumatoid and osteoarthritis, with a significant decrease in GI side effects.

(4) Ibuprofen has been shown to be equally efficacious as indomethacin in controlling symptoms of rheumatoid arthritis with a decreased incidence of GI side effects.

(5) Ibuprofen has been shown to be superior to propoxyphene in treating pain associated with episiotomy pain, pain associated with dental extractions, and primary dysmenorrhea.

(6) In patients with dysmenorrhea, ibuprofen has been shown to reduce prostaglandin activity in intrauterine fluid, directly reducing uterine contractions and decreasing intrauterine pressure.

(7) In children, 10 mg/kg of ibuprofen suspension has been shown to be as effective as 15 mg/kg of acetaminophen in reducing fever due to viral illness.

b. Pharmacokinetics

  (1) Absorption

    (a) Ibuprofen is rapidly absorbed from the GI tract with peak serum levels within 2 hours of oral administration.

    (b) Ibuprofen suspension is absorbed somewhat faster than in tablet form.

    (c) Co-ingestion of food may slightly slow absorption of ibuprofen but does not affect bioavailability; it may reduce the incidence of GI upset and is recommended for doses above 400 mg.

  (2) Metabolism

    (a) Ibuprofen is metabolized in the liver and excreted in the urine.

    (b) The serum half-life is 1.8 to 2 hours.

c. Administration and usage

  (1) Adult dosing:

    (a) Mild to moderate pain or fever: **400 mg every 4 to 6 hours** as necessary.

    (b) Dosages greater than 400 mg are no more effective than the 400-mg dose in acute pain.

    (c) Rheumatoid and osteoarthritis: **1200 to 3600 mg/day in divided doses** (400 mg, 600 mg, or 800 mg 3 or 4 times daily). Individual patients may respond better to 3200 mg/day, but exceeding 2400 mg has not shown a benefit in population studies and is associated with increased GI side effects.

  (2) Pediatric dosing:

    (a) Mild to moderate pain or fever: 5 to 10 mg/kg of ibuprofen suspension every 8 hours as needed

    (b) 5 mg/kg is recommended for fever reduction for temperatures < 102.5°

    (c) 10 mg/kg is recommended for fever reduction for temperatures > 102.5°

d. Contraindications and precautions:

  (1) Ibuprofen should not be administered to patients with a prior history of hypersensitivity to the drug.

(2) Ibuprofen should not be administered to patients with aspirin-sensitive asthma or the triad of asthma, nasal polyposis, and vasomotor rhinitis to avoid a potentially severe anaphylactoid reaction.

(3) **Ibuprofen, like all NSAIDs,** should be **used with caution** in patients with a preexisting **history of peptic ulcer disease or upper GI bleed, chronic renal insufficiency, or CHF and in patients taking ACE inhibitors, diuretics, glucocorticoids, oral anticoagulants, lithium, methotrexate, or phenytoin.**

e. Adverse effects

(1) Ibuprofen in doses of 800 to 1200 mg/day has a similar rate of GI side effects to acetaminophen.

(2) The most common adverse effect associated with ibuprofen use is dyspepsia.

(3) In clinical trials involving ibuprofen, the rate of GI side effects ranges from 4% to 16%.

(4) Ibuprofen has about half the rate of GI side effects of aspirin or indomethacin.

(5) Additional adverse effects are similar to those of all NSAIDs and were discussed previously.

f. Advantages

(1) Ibuprofen is an inexpensive, readily available analgesic, anti-inflammatory, and antipyretic.

(2) It has a favorable safety profile when compared with aspirin and has a low abuse liability.

g. Disadvantages

(1) Like all NSAIDs, ibuprofen has significant gastric toxicity and drug interactions.

(2) Standard dosing for ibuprofen is every 6 to 8 hours, as compared with every 8 to 12 hours for naproxen.

h. Clinical pearls

(1) Ibuprofen in doses of **400 mg** every 6 hours for adult patients or **10 mg/kg** in pediatric patients may be considered an alternative first-line medication to acetaminophen and an **NSAID of choice** for short-term treatment of mild to moderate acute pain owing to its extensively evaluated **safety profile.**

(2) Ibuprofen in doses of 800 to 1200 mg/day has a similar rate of GI side effects to acetaminophen.

(3) Ibuprofen in doses of 600 to 800 mg every 6 hours may be safely used in the short-term treatment of acute inflammatory pain, but longer-term usage is associated with increased GI side effects.

(4) **Ibuprofen, like all NSAIDs,** should be **used with caution** in patients with preexisting **history of peptic ulcer disease or upper GI bleed, chronic renal insufficiency, or CHF and in patients taking ACE inhibitors, diuretics, glucocorticoids, oral anticoagulants, lithium, methotrexate, or phenytoin.**

2. Naproxen
a. Overview:
  (1) Naproxen is a commonly administered NSAID of the aryl acetic acid class with analgesic, anti-inflammatory, and antipyretic properties.
  (2) It is available as **naproxen** (Naprosyn) in 250-, 375-, and 500-mg tablets and as a suspension containing 125 mg per 5 mL of naproxen.
  (3) Enteric-coated capsules are available containing 375 mg or 500 mg of naproxen.
  (4) It is also available as its sodium salt, **naproxen sodium** (Anaprox), for more rapid absorption in tablets containing 275 mg or 550 mg of naproxen sodium.
  (5) It is available over the counter as naproxen sodium 220 mg (Aleve) in tablets, caplets, and gel caplets.
  (6) Naproxen has been shown to be as effective as aspirin or indomethacin in the treatment of rheumatoid arthritis with fewer GI side effects.
  (7) Naproxen has been shown to be effective in reducing acute pain with onset of action within **1 hour with naproxen** and **30 minutes with naproxen sodium.**
b. Pharmacokinetics:
  (1) Absorption:
    (a) Peak plasma concentrations of **naproxen** are obtained in 2 to 3 hours after oral administration.
    (b) Peak plasma concentrations of **naproxen sodium** are obtained after 1 to 2 hours.
    (c) Naproxen delayed-released tablets yield peak plasma concentrations 4 to 6 hours after oral administration.
    (d) Once absorbed, naproxen is 99% bound to serum albumin.
  (2) Metabolism:
    (a) Naproxen is metabolized in the liver and excreted in the urine.
    (b) The plasma half-life ranges from 12 to 17 hours.
c. Dosing and administration:
  (1) Acute pain (analgesia, tendonitis, bursitis, or dysmenorrhea): Because of its more rapid absorption, **naproxen sodium** is recommended for acute pain with a starting dose of 550 mg followed by 550 mg every 12 hours or 275 mg every 6 to 8 hours as needed.
  (2) Acute gout:
    (a) The recommended starting dose is **500 mg of naproxen** followed by **250 mg** every 8 hours until the attack has subsided.
    (b) **Naproxen sodium** may be used in a dose of **550 mg** followed by **275 mg** every 8 hours as needed.
  (3) Osteoarthritis and rheumatoid arthritis:
    (a) 250 mg, 350 mg, or 500 mg of naproxen taken twice a day
    (b) 225 mg or 550 mg of naproxen sodium taken twice a day

(c) Total daily dose may be increased to 1500 mg/day for up to 6 months when a higher dose of anti-inflammatory activity is needed.

d. Contraindications and precautions:

(1) Naproxen or naproxen sodium should not be administered to a patient with a prior history of hypersensitivity to the drug.

(2) Naproxen should not be administered to patients with aspirin-sensitive asthma or the triad of asthma, nasal polyposis, and vasomotor rhinitis to avoid a potentially severe anaphylactoid reaction.

(3) **Naproxen, like all NSAIDs,** should be **used with caution** in patients with preexisting **history of peptic ulcer disease or upper GI bleed, chronic renal insufficiency, or CHF and in patients taking ACE inhibitors, diuretics, glucocorticoids, oral anticoagulants, lithium, methotrexate, or phenytoin.**

e. Adverse effects

(1) Like other NSAIDs, the most common adverse effect of naproxen is dyspepsia, occurring in 1% to 10% of patients who take the drug.

(2) Serious, life-threatening GI complications also occur with naproxen.

f. Advantages

(1) Inexpensive, effective, widely available analgesic, antipyretic, and anti-inflammatory drug, available over the counter as naproxen sodium, 220 mg, and in a wide range of prescription strengths.

(2) **Naproxen sodium** has a favorable pharmacodynamic profile when compared with ibuprofen (more rapid peak plasma levels, longer half-life) but the clinical relevance is unclear.

g. Disadvantages

(1) Less flexibility in dosing compared with ibuprofen.

(2) Naproxen has a longer onset of action compared with naproxen sodium and should not be a first-line agent for acute pain.

h. Clinical pearl: Naproxen sodium in doses of 550 mg may be considered a first-line medication for patients receiving an NSAID for acute pain who prefer **twice-daily dosage.**

3. Ketorolac

a. Overview

(1) **Ketorolac (Toradol)** is a member of the pyrrole group of NSAIDs with analgesic and anti-inflammatory properties and currently is the only parenteral NSAID available in the United States.

(2) Ketorolac is also available as an oral tablet for the short-term (up to 5 days) treatment of acute painful conditions that require analgesia at the opioid level. It is indicated only for continuation of parenteral ketorolac therapy. It is not recommended for mild to moderate pain or chronic painful conditions.

(3) Parenteral ketorolac has been shown to be an effective analgesic in a variety of acute pain states with a faster onset of action when compared with oral NSAIDs.

(4) IV ketorolac in a dose of 30 mg has been shown to have analgesic efficacy in the postoperative state between that of 6 mg and 12 mg of morphine.

(5) IV ketorolac in a dose of 30 mg has been shown to be as effective as 50 mg of meperidine in treating the pain associated with acute renal colic.

(6) Ketorolac has also been shown to have a similar efficacy to opioids in biliary colic and acute musculoskeletal pain.

(7) However, ketorolac has not been shown to be a more effective analgesic than ibuprofen in patients who are able to tolerate oral NSAIDs and offers little advantages with significantly higher cost in those patients.

b. Pharmacokinetics

  (1) **Onset:** Peak plasma concentrations are obtained at:

    (a) Approximately 40 minutes with oral administration

    (b) Approximately 30 minutes with intramuscular administration

    (c) Approximately 2 minutes with intravenous administration

    (d) Once absorbed, ketorolac is 99% bound to plasma albumin.

  (2) Half-life

    (a) In healthy individuals, the half-life is about 5 hours.

    (b) The half-life increases to 7 hours in elderly patients and 6 to 19 hours in patients with renal insufficiency.

  (3) **Elimination:** Ketorolac is metabolized in the liver and excreted in the urine as metabolites and as some unchanged drug.

c. Dosing and administration

  (1) **Single-dose treatment:** The following regimen should be limited to single administration use only:

    (a) IM

      (i) 60 mg IM in adults younger than 65 years

      (ii) 30 mg IM in adults older than 65 years, renally impaired, or less than 50 kg total body weight

      (iii) 1 mg/kg up to a total dose of 30 mg in pediatric patients aged 2 to 16 years

    (b) IV

      (i) 30 mg IV in adults younger than 65 years

      (ii) 15 mg IV in adults older than 65 years, renally impaired, or less than 50 kg total body weight

      (iii) 0.3–0.5 mg/kg up to 15 mg total dose in pediatric patients aged 2 to 16 years

  (2) Multiple-dose treatment (IV or IM) in adults

    (a) **Patients < 65 years of age:** The recommended dose is 30 mg Toradol IV/IM every 6 hours. The maximum daily dose should not exceed 120 mg.

    (b) **For patients ≥ 65 years of age, renally impaired patients, and patients weighing less than 50 kg (110 lb):** The recommended dose is 15 mg Toradol IV/IM every 6 hours.

The maximum daily dose for these populations should not exceed 60 mg.

   (c) For breakthrough pain, do not increase the dose or the frequency of Toradol. Consideration should be given to supplementing these regimens with low doses of opioids as needed unless otherwise contraindicated.

(3) Transition from Toradol IV/IM to Toradol PO in adults: The recommended Toradol oral dose is as follows:

   (a) **Patients < 65 years of age:** 2 tablets as a first oral dose for patients who received 60 mg IM single dose, 30 mg IV single dose, or 30 mg multiple dose. Toradol IV/IM followed by 1 tablet Toradol oral every 4 to 6 hours, not to exceed 30 mg/24 hours of Toradol oral.

   (b) **Patients ≥ 65 years of age, renally impaired, or weighing less than 50 kg (110 lb):** 1 tablet as a first oral dose for patients who received 30 mg IM single dose, 15 IV single dose, or 15 mg multiple dose. Toradol IV/IM followed by 1 tablet Toradol oral every 4 to 6 hours, not to exceed 20–30 mg/24 hours of Toradol oral. **Strongly consider an alternative agent in the patient groups.**

   (c) Shortening the recommended dosing intervals may result in increased frequency and severity of adverse reactions.

   (d) **In adults, the maximum combined duration of use (parenteral and oral Toradol) is limited to 5 days.**

d. Contraindications

   (1) Ketorolac should not be administered to patients with a prior history of hypersensitivity to the drug.

   (2) Ketorolac should not be administered to patients with aspirin-sensitive asthma or the triad of asthma, nasal polyposis, and vasomotor rhinitis to avoid a potentially severe anaphylactoid reaction.

   (3) **Ketorolac is only indicated for the short-term (up to 5 days in adults) management of moderately severe acute pain that requires analgesia at the opioid level. It is NOT indicated for minor or chronic painful conditions.**

   (4) **Ketorolac, like all NSAIDs,** should be **used with caution** in patients with preexisting **history of peptic ulcer disease or upper GI bleed, chronic renal insufficiency, or CHF and in patients taking ACE inhibitors, diuretics, glucocorticoids, oral anticoagulants, lithium, methotrexate, or phenytoin.**

e. Adverse effects: Ketorolac has significant GI and renal toxicity compared with other NSAIDs and is contraindicated for treatment of mild to moderate pain and for chronic conditions.

f. Advantages

   (1) Available for parenteral administration in patients who require analgesia at the opioid level who are unable to tolerate oral NSAIDs.

   (2) May have a more rapid onset of action than orally administered NSAIDs.

g. Disadvantages

   (1) More expensive than orally administered NSAIDs.

(2) Has not been shown to be more effective than orally administered NSAIDs.

(3) Requires administration by a trained individual.

(4) Significant GI and renal side effects limit duration of therapy to 5 days.

h. Clinical pearls

(1) Intravenous ketorolac may be used in patients whose nausea or vomiting precludes the oral administration of an NSAID, but it **has not been shown to be more efficacious** than oral NSAIDs in clinical practice.

(2) Ketorolac is **only** indicated for the **short-term** (up to 5 days in adults) management of moderately severe acute pain that requires analgesia at the opioid level. It is **NOT** indicated **for minor or chronic painful conditions.**

4. Indomethacin

a. Overview

(1) First approved by the FDA in 1964, indomethacin (Indocin) is an NSAID of the acetic acid group and is one of the oldest NSAIDs available in the United States.

(2) Indomethacin is a potent nonselective COX inhibitor and an effective analgesic, antipyretic, and anti-inflammatory agent; however, its increased incidence of GI side effects when compared with other NSAIDs makes indomethacin a poor choice for the first-line relief of acute pain.

(3) It is available as instant-release tablets, sustained-release capsules, oral suspension, and rectal suppositories.

b. Pharmacokinetics

(1) Onset

(a) After oral administration, indomethacin is readily absorbed, attaining peak plasma concentrations at about 2 hours.

(b) Orally administered indomethacin capsules are virtually 100% bioavailable, with 90% of the dose absorbed within 4 hours.

(c) Rectally administered suppositories have a more rapid absorption than oral tablets but a decreased bioavailability.

(d) Indomethacin extended-release capsules, 75 mg, are designed to release 25 mg of the drug initially and the remaining 50 mg over about 12 hours (90% of dose absorbed by 12 hours).

(2) Half-life: The mean half-life of indomethacin is estimated to be about 4.5 hours.

(3) Elimination

(a) Indomethacin is eliminated through renal excretion, metabolism, and biliary excretion.

(b) About 60% of an oral dosage is recovered in urine as drug and metabolites, and 33% is recovered in feces.

c. Indications and dosage: Indomethacin cannot be considered a simple analgesic and should not be used in conditions other than those recommended.

(2) Indications

   (a) Moderate to severe rheumatoid arthritis, including acute flares of chronic disease.

   (b) Moderate to severe ankylosing spondylitis; moderate to severe osteoarthritis

   (c) Acute painful shoulder (bursitis and/or tendonitis)

   (d) Acute gouty arthritis

(3) Dosages for acute pain

   (a) **Acute painful shoulder** (bursitis and/or tendonitis). Initial dose: 75 to 150 mg daily in 3 or 4 divided doses. The drug should be discontinued after the signs and symptoms of inflammation have been controlled for several days. The usual course of therapy is 7 to 14 days.

   (b) **Acute gouty arthritis.** Suggested dosage: Capsules—INDOCIN 50 mg, 3 times daily, until pain is tolerable. The dose should then be rapidly reduced to complete cessation of the drug. Definite relief of pain has been reported within 2 to 4 hours. Tenderness and heat usually subside in 24 to 36 hours, and swelling gradually disappears in 3 to 5 days.

d. Adverse effects

   (1) Indomethacin has shown about twice the rate of serious GI side effects as naproxen and ibuprofen.

   (2) It also has rates of symptomatic peptic ulcer disease similar to aspirin.

e. Advantages: Indomethacin has demonstrated no advantages over ibuprofen or naproxen in controlled clinical trials.

f. Disadvantages

   (1) Increased rate of serious GI side effects

   (2) Moderate incidence of headaches

   (3) Reported CNS complaints such as confusion. Mechanism is unclear.

g. Clinical pearl: Indomethacin has not conclusively been shown to be superior to other NSAIDs for any indication and may have a worse safety profile than other agents like ibuprofen. It does occupy a therapeutic niche for refractory pain in acute gouty arthritis, but the side-effect profile issues remain the same. Indomethacin therefore should not be considered a first-line drug for acute painful conditions.

VI. MUSCLE RELAXANTS

A. Introduction

1. The term *muscle relaxant* refers to a heterogeneous group of agents used clinically for either:

a. Upper motor neuron spasticity, *or*

b. Postinjury skeletal muscle pain and/or spasm

2. Examples of upper motor neuron (UMN) diagnoses encompassed by spinal cord reflex spasticity/spasm include:

a. Multiple sclerosis

b. Traumatic brain injury

c. Cerebrovascular accident
d. Spinal cord injury
3. FDA-approved muscle relaxants for UMN spasticity are:
a. Baclofen (Lioresal)
b. Tizanidine (Zanaflex)
c. Dantrolene (Dantrium)
d. All three of these agents are superior to placebo in improving tone and range of motion. Sparse data suggest that of the three, tizanidine may be slightly more efficacious.
4. Examples of "pure" skeletal muscle syndromes include:
a. Muscle strain
b. Radiculopathy with muscle spasm
c. Fibromyalgia
d. Cervicogenic headaches
e. Low back pain
5. For musculoskeletal pain, the agents shown in Table 2-1 are available.

B. Background

1. None of these agents actually work by modifying the membrane or motor end plate of skeletal muscle. In fact, it is likely that all exert their primary effect by CNS sedation with subsequent relaxation.
2. Caveats to this generalization are:
a. Baclofen acts at the spinal cord GABA B receptor and actually stimulates this inhibitory receptor both presynaptically and postsynaptically.
b. Diazepam acts at the spinal cord GABA A receptors in addition to its CNS sedative properties.
c. Dantrolene decreases calcium release from the intracellular sarcoplasmic reticulum and decreases the force of contraction of skeletal muscle.
d. The highest incidence of actual clinical **WEAKNESS** is seen with the baclofen.
e. Cyclobenzaprine may modulate spinal cord serotonin effects.

TABLE 2-1

MUSCLE RELAXANTS AVAILABLE FOR MUSCULOSKELETAL PAIN

Drug	$T_{1/2}$
Cyclobenzaprine (Flexeril)	2–3 hr
Methocarbamol (Robaxin)	1–2 hr
Metaxalone (Skelaxin)	2 hr
Orphenadrine (Norflex)	14 hr
Carisoprodol (Soma)	8 hr
Chlorzoxazone (Parafon Forte)	1–2 hr
Diazepam (Valium)	20–50 hr
Baclofen (Lioresal)	3 hr
Tizanidine (Zanaflex)	2.5 hr
Dantrolene (Dantrium)	3 hr

3. There is incredibly sparse data to suggest the superiority of any of these agents for musculoskeletal pain. This is particularly difficult because most acute pain syndromes are treated with a combination of narcotic and non-narcotic analgesics, physical therapy, and relaxants.
4. The few comparative trials available suggest that most of these relaxants are likely superior to placebo, and cyclobenzaprine may enjoy a slight efficacy superiority compared with the others.

C. Individual drug facts

1. Cyclobenzaprine (Flexeril)
a. FDA approved in 1977
b. May modulate serotonin receptors at the spinal cord level to modulate α-mononeuronal tone
c. May relieve spasm independent of sedation
d. Chemically very similar to amitriptyline
e. Potential for significant anticholinergic effects (glaucoma, supraventricular tachycardia (SVT), constipation, prostatism)
f. High degree of pain relief by 24 to 48 hours
g. Available as 5- and 10-mg tablets
h. Recommend starting at 5 mg PO 3 times daily. Escalate as needed to 10 mg PO 3 times daily.
2. Methocarbamol (Robaxin)
a. A CNS sedative chemically similar to guaifenesin
b. Poor data to argue for or against its use
c. Has been used in tetanus cases
d. Available as a parenteral form
e. 1 g/10 mL for IV or IM use
f. Tablet form: 500 mg, 750 mg
g. Dosage
    (1) 750 mg to 1500 mg PO 3 times daily
    (2) 1000 mg IM/IV 3 times daily × 48 hours
3. Metaxalone (Skelaxin)
a. FDA approved in 1964
b. No skeletal muscle effect
c. Moderate anticholinergic potential
d. Weak comparative clinical data
e. Primary side effects are sedation, nausea, and headache
f. Rare hypersensitivity reaction
g. Dosage: 400 to 800 mg PO 3 to 4 times daily
4. Orphenadrine (Norflex)
a. Derived from diphenhydramine
b. Minimal evidence for any skeletal muscle effect
c. Fair clinical analgesia
d. Analgesia may outweigh clinical muscle relaxant effects
e. Moderate anticholinergic potential
f. Available as parenteral form for IV/IM use

g. Dosage
  (1) 100 mg PO every 12 hours
  (2) 60 mg IV/IM every 12 hours
5. Carisoprodol (Soma)
a. FDA approved 1959 before updated rules for demonstrated efficacy
b. Active metabolite is meprobamate, an older-generation sedative
c. Carisoprodol has large abuse potential
d. Has been made a scheduled drug in some states (Schedule IV)
e. Its metabolite, meprobamate, is a scheduled drug.
f. Dosage: 350 mg PO 3 times daily
g. **Warning:** There is nothing to argue for the use of this drug over other muscle relaxants. Its relative position should make it the "meperidine of muscle relaxants"! (AUTHOR'S BIAS)
6. Chlorzoxazone (Parafon Forte)
a. Derivative of benzoxazolene
b. Renally excreted
c. Few comparative data
d. Rare hepatic injury
e. Rare spasmodic torticollis
f. Dosage: 250 to 750 mg PO 3 to 4 times daily
7. Baclofen (Lioresal)
a. Augments presynaptic and postsynaptic GABA B receptors
b. Also FDA approved for intrathecal use for spasticity (through continuous infusion pump)
c. Analgesic potential with neuropathic pain syndromes
d. Beware toxicity with renal insufficiency
e. Clinical weakness can be an issue
f. Beware abrupt withdrawal with higher doses
g. Dosage
  (1) Start 10 mg PO 3 times daily
  (2) Advance 5 to 10 mg every 2 to 3 days
  (3) Maximum ± 60 to 80 mg/day
8. Tizanidine (Zanaflex)
a. A centrally acting α_2 agonist (e.g., clonidine)
b. Equivalent to baclofen, but with lower rates of weakness
c. Has a reasonable track record for headache and UMN muscle pain syndromes
d. Significant chance of hypotension and orthostasis
e. Must be slowly titrated
f. Dosage
  (1) 4 mg PO 3 times daily
  (2) Advance to maximum 32 mg/day
9. Dantrolene (Dantrium)
a. Blocks intracellular calcium mobilization from sarcoplasmic reticulum
b. Main utilization has been with malignant hyperthermia and some cases of neuroleptic malignant syndrome. Parenteral use in these cases is necessary.

c. Beware possible hepatic damage
d. Not a first-line drug for typical musculoskeletal pain syndromes
e. Dosage
    (1) Start 25 mg PO 4 times daily
    (2) Advance as needed to 100 mg PO 2 to 3 times daily

D. Final caveats

1. Muscle relaxants are indicated for either UMN spasticity or acute musculoskeletal injury.
2. Muscle relaxants are not really muscle relaxants. They do not work (with the possible exception of dantrolene) at the striated muscle. Sedation is an important component of their action.
3. Baclofen, diazepam, and tizanidine affect muscle tone through a spinal cord action.
4. Some muscle relaxants appear to have an actual analgesic effect. Examples are baclofen, tizanidine, and perhaps cyclobenzaprine.
5. Cyclobenzaprine has the strongest data support for efficacy among the non-UMN muscle relaxants. A dose of 5 mg may be as effective as the 10 mg dose.
6. Beware excessive sedation and anticholinergic effects from muscle relaxants.
7. Muscle relaxants should almost always be part of a comprehensive regimen that includes NSAIDs, analgesics, and possibly physical therapy.

BIBLIOGRAPHY

Beebe FA, Barkin RL, Barkin S. A clinical and pharmacologic review of skeletal muscle relaxants for musculoskeletal conditions. *Am J Ther* 2005; 12(2):151–171.

Chou R, Peterson K, Helfand M. Comparative efficacy and safety of skeletal muscle relaxants for spasticity and musculoskeletal conditions: A systematic review of pain symptom management. *J Pain Symptom Manage* 2004; 28(2):140–175.

Crofford LJ. Nonsteroidal anti-inflammatory drugs. In Harris (ed), *Kelley's Textbook of Rheumatology*, 7th ed. Philadelphia: Elsevier, 2006.

Fosnocht DE. Changing attitudes about pain and pain control in emergency medicine. *Emerg Med Clin North Am* 2005; 23(2):297–306.

Innes GD. Basic pharmacology and advances in emergency medicine. *Emerg Med Clin North Am* 2005; 23(2):433–465, ix–x.

Kijur PE. Intravenous morphine at 0.1 mg/kg is not effective for controlling severe acute pain in the majority of patients. *Ann Emerg Med* 2005; 46(4):362–367.

Lee MA. Retrospective study of the use of hydromorphone in palliative care patients with normal and abnormal urea and creatinine. *Palliat Med* 2001; 15(1):26–34.

Toth PP, Urtis J. Commonly used muscle relaxant therapies for acute low back pain: A review of carisoprodol, cyclobenzaprine hydrochloride, and metaxalone. *Clin Ther* 2004; 26(9):1355–1367.

Opioid Tolerance, Dependence, and Withdrawal: Recognition and Treatment

W. James Phillips and Anna Lerant

I. BACKGROUND

A. Opiates

1. Opiates exert their effect through a complex interaction with three specific receptor types: mu (μ), delta (δ), and kappa (κ). These are G-protein–coupled receptors that act by decreasing cyclic AMP (cAMP) levels or by activating an ion channel (potassium).
2. Changes in intracellular cAMP predict many cellular changes, including tolerance and physical dependence. Opiates also decrease calcium ion entry (which diminishes presynaptic neuronal activity) and increase potassium ion efflux (which hyperpolarizes postsynaptic neurons). A γ-aminobutyric acid (GABA) action is also likely (Figs. 3-1 and 3-2).
3. Opiate receptors are located in the cortex, thalamus, midbrain, spinal cord, and even peripheral tissues (particularly after inflammation or injury). Pure agonist agents (morphine-like) work primarily at the μ receptor, compared with agonist-antagonist agents, which are likely agonist at the κ receptor but antagonist at the μ receptor.
4. The euphoric and rewarding properties of opiates are likely mediated through the mesolimbic dopamine system.

B. Tolerance

1. Physiologic tolerance is a profound decrease in the analgesic effect during prolonged administration of an opiate at a given dose. It eventually occurs in all patients, but at different rates based on clinical observation.
2. Tolerance presents as escalating dose requirements, typically in the face of clinically static pain problems. One must be extremely careful not to confuse tolerance with increased pain from disease progression (malignancies with growth or metastases) or a change in the pain diagnosis (e.g., new radiculopathy, hematoma, or fracture development).

C. Cellular changes

1. Potential mechanisms for the development of tolerance include:
a. Receptor down-regulation (decreased number)
b. Receptor desensitization (decreased receptor reactivity)

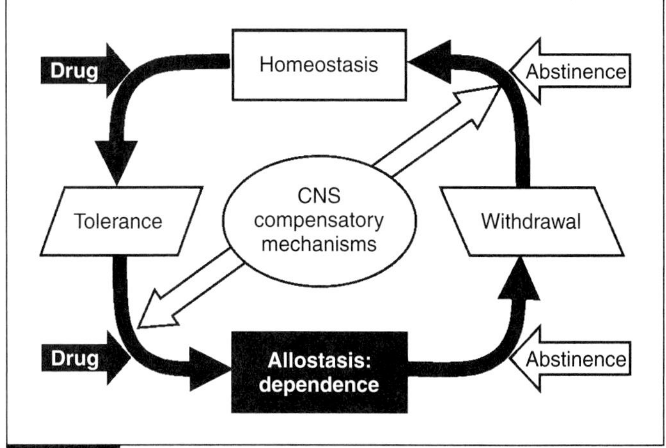

FIG. 3-1

Events of chronic opiate administration and withdrawal. Dependence develops as a result of gradually increasing compensatory mechanisms in the brain's reward system. Compensatory mechanisms "tune" pain perception and reward system to an allostatic state, **addiction,** when the patient is unable to function without opiates present. Opiate **abstinence** leads to dramatic **withdrawal signs,** which subside with maintained abstinence. As compensatory mechanisms allow recovery of the reward system, the patient returns to physiologic pain sensitivity.

    c. Uncoupling from downstream pain pathways
    d. Receptor reserve pool changes
  2. Positive and negative changes in receptor density have been observed during chronic opiate treatment. Tolerance may also develop in vivo with no change in receptor density.
  3. Actual receptor desensitization may occur within minutes to hours, followed in days to weeks by the development of clinical tolerance. The degree of receptor desensitization may vary widely according to the location of the receptor in the nervous system.
    a. Example: Clinical tolerance develops readily in areas mediating nociception and respiratory depression/sedation, but very little in areas mediating the euphoric/reinforcing (dependence) or constipating effect.
    b. This desensitization is likely a G-protein–uncoupling phenomenon.
  4. Following chronic opiate treatment, intracellular cAMP levels are elevated. This implies that although opiate occupancy of cell surface receptors is unchanged, the ability of the receptors to decrease cAMP levels has been lost or diminished.
  5. Opiate receptors are continually recycled. Receptors that have been occupied or stimulated for some period of time undergo endocytosis and

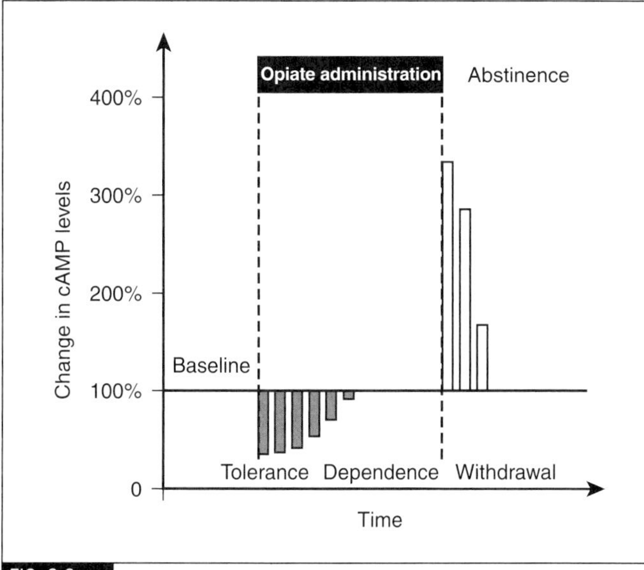

FIG. 3-2

Cyclic adenosine monophosphate (cAMP) levels in μ-opiate administration over time. Acute administration of opioid agonists causes a significant decrease in intracellular cAMP levels, promoting hyperpolarization of the neuron and resulting in analgesia. Continued opioid administration activates intracellular signals, which gradually diminish μ-opiate agonist-induced decreases in the cAMP levels. Development of opiate tolerance over time correlates with the gradual return of intracellular cAMP levels to baseline, despite sustained opiate administration. In opiate-dependent patients, opioid administration is necessary to keep cAMP levels at baseline and prevent withdrawal-induced pain. (*Data from Meyer JS, Quenzer LF: Psychopharmacology: Drugs, the Brain, and Behavior. Sunderland, MA, Sinauer Associates, 2005.*)

"intracellular recycling." Theoretically, more efficacious (i.e., lipophilic) opiates that exert their effect while occupying fewer receptors may leave a larger pool of receptors (reserve pool) unoccupied for later stimulation during subsequent drug dosing (Fig. 3-3).

II. TREATMENT OF OPIATE TOLERANCE

A. Once tolerance begins to develop, there are several choices, none of which is optimal or guaranteed efficacious. These are:
1. Dose escalation
2. Opiate rotation
3. Addition of co-analgesics
4. Initiate more invasive techniques

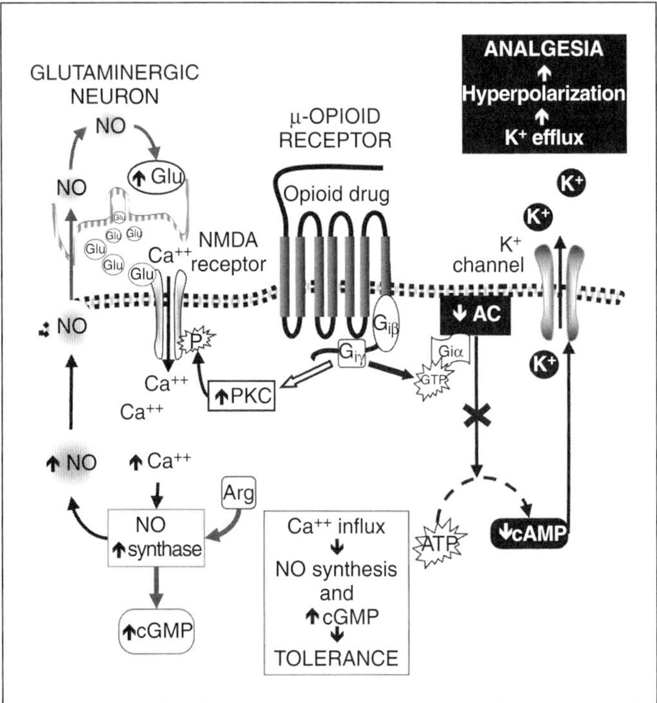

FIG. 3-3

Signaling pathways activated by ligand binding to μ-opioid receptors. Analgesia: The μ-opioid receptors are G-protein coupled seven transmembrane receptors. Upon ligand binding to opiate receptors, the inhibitory Giα component dissociates from the Gi-protein heterotrimer and decreases adenylate cyclase (AC) enzyme activity. Lower AC activity results in decreased intracellular cyclic adenosine monophosphate (cAMP) levels, which activate the K+ channels. Increased K+ permeability leads to K+ efflux from the neuron and **hyperpolarization.** In hyperpolarization, the chance of action potential generation decreases, and the pain transmission pathway is interrupted, leading to analgesia. **Tolerance:** Sustained activation of μ-opioid receptors activate protein kinase C (PKC) enzyme in the neuron. PKC phosphorylates the NMDA glutamate receptors, increasing the influx of Ca++ into the cell. Increased intracellular Ca++ concentrations activate the nitric oxide (NO) synthase (NOS) enzyme, resulting in increased NO and cyclic guanosine monophosphate (cGMP) levels. NO, a gaseous neurotransmitter, diffuses into presynaptic glutaminergic neurons, leading to sustained glutamate release and excitatory input to the neuron. cGMP also promotes intracellular events, which lower the threshold of action potential formation in the neuron. Chronic activation of μ receptors by both endogenous (dynorphin) and exogenous agonists may cause **opiate-induced pain.**

B. Increase the dose of the current opiate—this effectively serves to saturate the target receptor population. This dose escalation may buy time, but tolerance to the new dose is relatively inevitable.

C. Opioid rotation involves changing to a totally new opiate. Although scientific data are scant, much clinical associated evidence supports this practice. As with variability in individual responses to nonsteroidal anti-inflammatory drugs (NSAIDs), there is likely significant individual variability in response to different opiates, even though all the agents work at the same receptor complex.
1. Incomplete cross-tolerance is observed for many of the opiates, with methadone being the best example.
a. Practically, this means that when switching from one opiate to another, it is prudent to start at a lower dose than that calculated from the "equi-analgesic bibles" (which are based on single dose efficiency!).
b. Typically, opiate rotation schemes will start at one half to one third the calculated equi-analgesic 24-hour dose.
c. Example:
    (1) Current patient regimen = meperidine, 400 mg/24 hours
    (2) Rotate to morphine: 400 mg meperidine = 40 mg morphine (morphine is 10 times as potent as meperidine)
    (3) 40 mg morphine × **"incomplete cross-tolerance factor"**
    (4) 0.66 = 25 mg morphine (some authors recommend reduction by 50% rather than 33% and then titrating up)
    (5) New 24-hour total = morphine sulfate, 25 mg

D. Drug combination may potentially enhance analgesia, reduce side effects, and help reduce the rate of opiate dose escalation. Drug combinations should be carefully tailored to the individual patient, taking into account side effects, organ toxicity, sedative properties, and anticipated duration of pain (Table 3-1).

E. When oral or parenteral opioids or co-analgesics fail to adequately treat the pain, more invasive techniques should be considered. These might include:
1. Peripheral nerve blockade by continuous infusion (brachial plexus, femoral nerve)
2. Continuous epidural catheter infusion for 3 to 5 days
3. Placement of an indwelling intrathecal infusion system (which is typically reserved for cancer pain)
4. Consultation for ablative or neurolytic techniques:
a. Celiac plexus block for abdominal cancer
b. Hypogastric plexus block for pelvic cancer

III. DEPENDENCE

A. Dependence may be physical or psychological. Physical dependence is manifested by the presence of a withdrawal syndrome upon

TABLE 3-1

CO-ANALGESIC EXAMPLES

Agent	24-Hour Dose	Elimination Route	Side Effects	Co-analgesic Mechanism	Half-Life	Caveats
Acetaminophen	Max: 4 g	Hepatic	Hepatic	CNS prostagland in central modulation	4 hr	Beware total acetaminophen dose in drug combination
Aspirin	Max: 3 g	Hepatic	Hepatic, renal, and GI	Peripheral prostagland in modulation	4 hr	Beware platelet dysfunction and salicylate toxicity syndrome
COX inhibitors (NSAIDs)	Variable	Renal, hepatic	Hepatic, renal, and GI	Peripheral prostaglandin modulation	Variable	COX-2 inhibitors *not* proven as better analgesics than COX-1 inhibitors; beware cardiac issues
Antihistamines	25–50 mg every 8 hr	Hepatic	Sedation	Sedation anxiolysis	6 hr	Hydroxyzine has best record as co-analgesic
Dextro-amphetamine (Dexedrine)	2.5–10 mg, 3 times a day	Hepatic	Euphoria, sleep disruption	CNS catecholamine modulation	Variable	Avoid evening doses; useful to combat opiate sedation; use drug holidays
Methylphenidate (Ritalin)	5–10 mg, 3 times a day	Renal, hepatic	Euphoria, sleep disruption	CNS catecholamine modulation	Variable	Avoid evening doses; useful to combat opiate sedation; use drug holidays; available as sustained release
Nortriptyline (Pamelor)	25–150 mg every bedtime	Hepatic	Sedation, anticholinergic effects	CNS catechol modulation (more norepinephrine)	Variable	Typically used every night; start at 25 mg/day; increase by 25 mg every 3–7 days; fewer anticholinergic effects

Amitriptyline (Elavil)	25–150 mg every night	Hepatic	Sedation, anticholinergic effects	CNS catechol modulation (more serotonin)	Variable	Metabolized to nortriptyline; more anticholinergic effects
Gabapentin	300–3000 mg divided 3 times daily	Hepatic, renal	Sedation, ataxia	N-type Ca channel modulation "membrane stabilization" **(developed as GABA agonist, but does not directly act at this receptor)**	8–12 hr	Least sedating of anticonvulsants; good margin of safety; better tolerated by elderly patients. Adjust dose for lower Creatinine Clearance (CRCL)
Bisphosphonates	Variable	Renal	GI, renal	Best for bone pain, neuropathic pain	Variable	Lower escalation schedule and target dose in elderly "niche" is for neuropathic pain like TCA
Corticosteroids	Variable	Hepatic	Hypertension, elevated glucose, peptic ulcer disease, weight gain, infection	Neuronal modulation, anti-inflammatory, sense of well-being	Variable	Decadron useful parenterally; prednisone usually preferred PO; taper as rapidly as possible; should provide GI protection: H_2 blocker, proton pump inhibitor

CNS, central nervous system; COX, cyclooxygenase; GABA, γ-aminobutyric acid; GI, gastrointestinal.

abrupt discontinuation. Patients with psychological dependence may manifest this dependence in the absence of physical dependence; most patients with physical dependence do not have psychological dependence.

B. Actual addiction is quite rare in patients treated with appropriate doses of analgesics for legitimate pain problems.

C. Physical dependence occurs at different rates with different individuals. Anecdotally, one should consider the possibility of withdrawal symptoms in patients receiving regularly scheduled opiates for longer than several weeks. The appearance of tolerance should raise the question of the possibility of withdrawal occurring if medications are abruptly stopped.

D. The time course of the withdrawal syndrome (salivation, lacrimation, nausea, vomiting, abdominal cramps, myoclonus, and agitation) is variable but typically begins within 6 to 12 hours and peaks at 24 to 72 hours. Withdrawal symptoms may be delayed 2 to 3 days after long-acting agents such as methadone.

E. Appearance of withdrawal syndrome requires:
1. Usually hospitalization
2. Reinitiation of opiate therapy
3. Treatment of autonomic hyperactivity with antihypertensives (clonidine and/or α and β blockers)
4. Slow and gradual drug tapering—generally 10% reduction every 1 to 3 days
5. Central α agonists may be useful adjuncts to help control agitation and autonomic hyperactivity

IV. ESOTERIC INTRAVENOUS REGIMENS

A. Overview

Intravenous infusion therapy has been described for a number of classes of agents. This technique may be tried in a number of situations, such as:
1. Diagnostic infusion for specific pain syndromes, such as a sympathetically mediated pain or complex regional pain syndrome.
2. A diagnostic infusion to try and assess whether a pain syndrome has neuropathic components. Some intravenous agents, as a clinical observation, appear to achieve more results in cases of neuropathic pain.
3. A pretest before considering a trial of an oral agent that acts by the same mechanism.
4. An alternative analgesic pathway when more traditional techniques fail.
5. Specific treatments for well-defined conditions, such as bisphosphonates for bone pain due to metastatic cancer.

Note: *A clinical observation has been that in some cases, the analgesic effect from a parenteral agent may far outlast the expected half-life of the administered drug.*

B. Pain conditions that may be amenable to infusion therapy
1. Neuropathic pain syndromes
a. These include:
   (1) Spinal cord injury pain
   (2) Peripheral neuropathy
   (3) Trigeminal neuropathy
   (4) Postherpetic neuralgia
   (5) Post-stroke pain
   (6) Sympathetically mediated pain
b. Potentially useful agents
   (1) Lidocaine
      (a) An amide local anesthetic that acts by modulating voltage-dependent sodium channels. Lidocaine is one of those agents that may have unique analgesic potential for neuropathic pain.
      (b) The intent is to infuse a generous but hopefully not toxic (seizure, cardiac arrest) dose over about 1 hour.
      (c) Technique
         (i) 500 mL intravenous fluid (IVF) preload.
         (ii) Continuous blood pressure and cardiac monitoring.
         (iii) 4 to 5 mg/kg preservative-free lidocaine infused over 60 minutes.
         (iv) When the patient experiences mild local anesthetic effect (e.g., dysarthria, tinnitus, circumoral), assess for analgesia from the pain distribution in question.
         (v) A response to intravenous lidocaine may predict a possible benefit from oral mexiletine, an orally available lidocaine analogue (antiarrhythmic).
   (2) Phentolamine
      (a) A peripherally acting α_1-receptor blocker that antagonizes the effect of synaptically released norepinephrine.
      (b) It may be somewhat specific for sympathetic nervous system synapses, but this is unclear. It may be beneficial not only for sympathetically mediated pain (visceral-renal colic, pancreatitis, or limbic pain) but also for large fiber neuropathic pain when damaged fibers have developed abnormal synaptic connections with the efferent sympathetic nervous system.
      (c) Technique
         (i) IVF 500 mL preload.
         (ii) Continuous noninvasive cardiac monitor.
         (iii) Consider propranolol, 1 mg IV, for reflex tachycardia. Metoprolol, 5 mg IV, is an alternative.
         (iv) Infuse phentolamine, 0.5–1 mg/kg over 30 minutes, and assess pain scores.
         (v) Patients may anticipate a modest vasodilatory headache and mild nasal congestion.
         (vi) Beware of hypotension.

(3) Adenosine
  (a) Although primarily an antiarrhythmic, adenosine receptors are also located on the spinal cord dorsal horn and possibly on peripheral nerves.
  (b) Technique
    (i) Continuous cardiac monitoring
    (ii) Adenosine, 50 µg/kg/min over 45 to 60 minutes
(4) Magnesium
  (a) Acts as an *N*-methyl-D-aspartate (NMDA) antagonist and has been used in neuropathic pain syndromes and for vascular headaches (migraines).
  (b) The dose is 20 to 30 mg/kg IV over 1 to 2 hours.
  (c) Beware neuromuscular depression and **clinical weakness.**
  (d) Beware vasodilation and hypotension.
(5) Ketamine
  (a) Not only a profound NMDA antagonist, but it also modulates calcium and sodium channels. Although used primarily for central and peripheral neuropathic pain syndromes, it may also be useful for:
    (i) Postoperative pain
    (ii) Chronic visceral pain
    (iii) Musculoskeletal pain when traditional opioids or NSAIDs are insufficient
    (iv) **Cases of opioid tolerance**

Note: *Psychomimetic side effects may be significant. These may be reduced by co-administration of benzodiazepines.*

  (b) Technique
    (i) Consider preprocedure midazolam
    (ii) Continuous cardiac monitoring with pulse oximetry
    (iii) Ketamine bolus, 0.1 to 0.3 mg/kg
    (iv) Ketamine infusion, 3 to 6 µg/kg/min for 30 to 60 minutes

Caveat: *Avoid in patients with any psychiatric history.*

2. Chronic abdominal pain
a. Octreotide is a somatostatin analogue that has been observed to have a potential effect in cases of visceral pain. Dose ranges are 100 to 600 µg IV or SC daily.
b. Phentolamine: since visceral pain is largely mediated with/through the afferent sympathetic/splanchnic system, modulation of this transmission or interruption of the ongoing sensitization may be possible.
c. Phentolamine has been described for renal colic, pancreatitis pain, cyclic vomiting syndrome, and the pain of pancreatic carcinoma.

3. Peripheral ischemic pain

a. As seen with ischemic peripheral neuropathy, vasculitis, or arterial insufficiency. This may be amenable to modulation by sympathetic nervous system interruption with phentolamine.

b. A successful trial may signal a possible benefit from an oral α-blocker therapy.

4. Opioid tolerance

a. In cases of chronic pain flares in the opioid tolerant, an opioid rotation technique with infusion of a highly lipophilic opioid may be undertaken.

b. Choices of lipophilic opioids include, in descending order of potency:

(1) Remifentanil, 1 to 2 µg/kg/hour

(2) Alfentanil, 20 to 40 µg/kg/hour

(3) Fentanyl, 3 to 5 µg/kg/hour

c. A 1- to 2-hour infusion may provide analgesia when current opioid effects have waned.

d. Beware: Respiratory depression, hypoxemia, synergistic sedation with other agents, and chest wall rigidity.

5. Bone pain from metastases

a. The bisphosphonates may be acutely and chronically useful. The mechanism of the acute analgesia is unclear. The mechanism of the chronic analgesia is inhibition of osteoclast activity.

b. Technique

(1) Pamidronate: 15 to 30 mg IV over 2 hours; may be repeated every 1 to 2 weeks

(2) Caveat

(a) Use of these techniques has often been based on small series or case reports.

(b) Many of these infusion techniques are with agents not commonly used by nonanesthesiologists or other specialists.

(c) At a minimum, awareness of their application would enable appropriate consultation and potential application when needed.

V. FINAL CAVEATS

A. Tolerance may develop within days.

B. Do not confuse tolerance with disease progression.

C. Tolerance to an opiate does not portend tolerance to a different opiate.

D. When utilizing an opiate rotation technique, decrease the starting daily dose by one third to one half to account for incomplete cross-tolerance.

E. IV infusion therapies may be applicable in cases of refractory pain or acute flares of chronic pain, and as a diagnostic maneuver, particularly when the sympathetic nervous system is suspected to be playing a role.

BIBLIOGRAPHY

Grabow T. Intravenous drug infusions. In Staats P, Wallace M (eds), *Pain Medicine and Management: Just the Facts*. New York: McGraw-Hill, 2005: 296–301.

Inturrisi C. Clinical pharmacology of opioids for pain. *Clin J Pain* 2002; 18:s3–s13.

Waldhoer M, Bartlett S, Whistler J. Opioid receptors. *Ann Rev Biochem* 2004; 73:953–990.

Acute Pain Management in the Chronic Pain Patient

W. James Phillips

I. BACKGROUND

A. There is an increasing tendency to prescribe opiates on a chronic basis for nonmalignant pain syndromes. Such patients may be maintained on a chronic daily regimen of opiate analgesics, the drug levels of which address the *chronic* pain problem but provide minimal analgesia for the *acute, new,* or *additional* pain.

B. Most patients on chronic opiates are using the drugs correctly and legitimately. Indeed, the incidence of *addiction* is probably no higher in the chronic pain population than in the general population (5% to 18%).

C. Key to successful treatment of these patients is appreciating that drug *tolerance* does not equate to *addiction*. Relevant terms for familiarization are:

1. *Addiction*: a compulsive preoccupation with and continued use of an agent despite no benefit and often in the face of harmful effects
2. *Psychological dependence*: the need for a psychoactive agent for its positive CNS effects or to avoid negative effects from withdrawal
3. *Physical dependence*: a physiologic state wherein a withdrawal syndrome occurs during abstinence
4. *Tolerance*: when more drug is required to produce a desired effect
a. Tolerance may be pharmacokinetic or pharmacodynamic.
b. Pharmacokinetic tolerance is generally due to hepatic enzyme induction and essentially cross-tolerance with drugs such as alcohol, barbiturates, or antiepileptics.
c. Pharmacodynamic tolerance reflects what takes place at the receptor or cellular level with:
   (1) Decrease in receptor density or uncoupling of receptors from G proteins
   (2) Up-regulation of the cyclic adenosine monophosphate (cAMP) pathway (normally inhibited by opiates)
   (3) Activation of *N*-methyl-D-aspartate (NMDA) receptors
d. Of note, clinical tolerance may last for months or years after discontinuation of the inciting drug.

II. MANAGEMENT

A. The first step in acute pain relief in the opiate-tolerant patient is calculating the historical "basal" opiate requirements and appreciating that this amount of drug does little to provide any acute analgesia for any new pain.

B. This amount of drug must be provided as a baseline.
C. The next step is initiating a plan for acute pain management of the "new" pain.
D. Options may include:
1. Initially make the patient comfortable and assess acute analgesia requirements by parenteral titration of morphine, hydromorphone, or fentanyl.
2. If the patient can take oral medications, continue the long-acting opiate such as morphine sulfate (MS) Contin or OxyContin twice daily supplemented with shorter-acting agents for the new pain.
a. That is, MS Contin twice daily with oxycodone, *or*
b. Hydrocodone every 4 to 6 hours for added analgesia
3. If the patient is unable to take oral medication, AFTER ANALGESIC TITRATION TO COMFORT, initiate a basal infusion of morphine or hydromorphone to cover the maintenance 24-hour drug requirements with a patient-controlled analgesia (PCA) technique for acute pain management.
a. That is, a patient taking MS Contin, 30 mg twice daily chronically sustains a femur fracture.
b. Daily morphine requirements = 60 mg orally = 20 mg IV, so
c. Basal infusion of morphine 0.8 mg/hour with a PCA dose of 2 mg IV every 5 to 10 minutes for the femur fracture pain.
4. As above, when converting from oral to parenteral medications, remember the effect of hepatic first-pass clearance. Conversion ratio from oral to parenteral:
a. Morphine = 3:1 oral to IV
b. Hydromorphone = 2:1 oral to IV
c. OxyContin has excellent oral bioavailability but no parenteral form. A possible conversion plan would be:
   (1) Chronic dose of 40 mg OxyContin per day
   (2) 40 mg OxyContin = 40 mg morphine (1:1 conversion)
   (3) **Because it has no significant first-pass effect,** 40 mg OxyContin PO per day = 40 mg IV morphine/day
5. Remember methadone may have incomplete cross-tolerance with other opiates and may be an excellent option. Methadone is available orally and for parenteral use. Conversion ratios may vary, but a useful starting conversion would be:
a. 10 mg morphine = 3 to 5 mg methadone
b. Example: patient taking MS Contin, 30 mg PO twice daily = 60 mg/day
   (1) Methadone substitution = 10 mg, 2 to 3 times daily
   (2) = roughly 30 mg/day
c. For patients with inadequate analgesia from parenteral morphine, a methadone PCA may be tried with bolus doses of 1.25 to 2.5 mg every 15 to 30 minutes.

6. Maximize the use of regional anesthesia techniques (typically requiring anesthesiology consultation). Examples include:
a. Brachial plexus blockade and/or catheter placement for upper extremity pain.
b. Continuous epidural catheter infusions of opiates and dilute local anesthetics.
c. Femoral nerve or lumbar plexus blockade or catheter placement for femur or lower extremity pain.
7. Maximize the use of co-analgesics, such as:
a. Nonsteroidal anti-inflammatory drugs (NSAIDs): Obviously most indicated for acute inflammation. Beware renal, gastrointestinal, and cardiac side effects (fluid retention, hyperkalemia).
b. "Neuropathic pain": Agents such as the anticonvulsants or tricyclic antidepressants. Recall that these agents must generally be titrated upward and are therefore less useful for acute pain.
c. Ketamine is probably underutilized as an opiate-sparing analgesic. Low-dose basal infusions of 5 to 15 mg/hour may provide excellent short-term supplemental analgesia with few psychomimetic side effects.
8. "Weaning": Once the new or acute pain issue has subsided or has been treated, it will be necessary to gradually titrate down the recent additions in opiates provided.
a. This should generally be done over 7 to 14 days with reduction of about 10% a day.
b. Reductions are done by downward titration of short-acting opiates such as hydrocodone or oxycodone **after reinstating** the preinjury longer-acting opiate regimen, that is, MS Contin, OxyContin, methadone, or fentanyl patches.

BIBLIOGRAPHY

Bloodworth D. Opioids in the treatment of chronic pain: Legal framework and therapeutic indication and limitations. *Phys Med Rehabil Clin N Am* 2006; 17(2):353–381.
Mitra S, Sinatra RS. Perioperative management in the opioid dependent patient. *Anesthesiology* 2004; 101:212–227.

Procedural Sedation

W. James Phillips and Anna Lerant

I. PROCEDURAL SEDATION: JOINT COMMISSION ON ACCREDITATION OF HEALTH CARE ORGANIZATIONS (JCAHO) POLICY AND REALITY

A. JCAHO defines levels of sedation:

1. *Minimal sedation (anxiolysis)*: a medically induced state during which patients respond normally to verbal commands. Cognitive function and coordination may be impaired; ventilatory and cardiovascular systems are unaffected.

2. *Moderate sedation/analgesia (conscious sedation)*: a drug-induced depression of consciousness during which patients respond purposefully to verbal commands, either alone or accompanied by light tactile stimulation. No interventions are required to maintain a patent airway, and spontaneous ventilation is adequate. Cardiovascular function is usually maintained.

3. *Deep sedation/analgesia*: a drug-induced depression of consciousness during which patients cannot easily be aroused but respond purposefully following repeated or painful stimulation. The ability to independently maintain ventilatory function may be impaired. Patients undergoing deep sedation have a significant risk for partial or complete loss of protective reflexes, including the ability to consistently maintain a patent airway independently and the inability to respond purposefully to physical stimulation or verbal commands. Loss of gag reflex, inability to handle oral secretions, and loss of swallowing reflex may occur. Patients may require assistance in maintaining a patent airway, and spontaneous ventilation may be inadequate. Cardiovascular function is maintained.

4. *Anesthesia*: consists of general anesthesia and spinal or major regional anesthesia. It does not include local anesthesia. General anesthesia is a drug-induced loss of consciousness during which patients are not arousable, even by painful stimulation. The ability to independently maintain ventilatory function is often impaired. Patients often require assistance in maintaining a patent airway, and positive pressure ventilation may be required because of depressed spontaneous ventilation or drug-induced depression of neuromuscular function. Cardiovascular function may be impaired.

B. Reality

1. You need to think in terms of *procedural* sedation, in which you balance the *individual needs* of the patient (anxiety level, perceived pain thresholds) with the *degree of pain* anticipated

from the procedures with the *cardiopulmonary status* of the patient.

2. **Caveat #1:** Every "sedation" case is a potential anemic, hypotensive patient requiring ventilatory assistance, airway management, and blood pressure resuscitation.

3. **Caveat #2**

a. Do not embark on procedural sedation if you don't have:
   (1) Full airway gear
   (2) Suction
   (3) Positive pressure oxygen
   (4) Resuscitation drugs
   (5) Full American Society of Anesthesiology (ASA) monitors
   (6) A **competent** assistant

b. And if you cannot:
   (1) Recognize cardiopulmonary insufficiency
   (2) Mask ventilate
   (3) Intubate well
   (4) Use resuscitation drugs
   (5) Call for reliable help

c. And if you have not:
   (1) Fully evaluated the patient
   (2) Assessed the airway
   (3) Noted pertinent history
   (4) Documented everything
   (5) Tailored the sedation plan to that patient's condition and status!

d. If you violate any of these rules, you may be **unsafe.**

4. **Caveat #3:** You must be credentialed in your hospital (Fig. 5-1).

a. You must demonstrate training.

b. You must demonstrate airway and drug competencies.

c. You must be ACLS qualified.

d. You must be signed off by your chairman.

II. PREPROCEDURE EVALUATION

A. Every institution will have a standard form.

1. See Figure 5-2 for an example.

2. This will guide you through key questions and pertinent physical examination areas you should evaluate.

B. As you evaluate the patient, you should be constantly asking yourself if you can manage the airway in an emergency.

1. Pertinent highlights:

a. NPO status

b. Cardiopulmonary history and current status

c. Medications, concurrent sedatives, analgesics

d. Airway

THE UNIVERSITY OF MISSISSIPPI MEDICAL CENTER
THE UNIVERSITY HOSPITALS AND CLINICS
JACKSON, MISSISSIPPI

DELINEATION OF CLINICAL or PRACTICE PRIVILEGES
PROCEDURAL SEDATION for NON-ANESTHESIA

_______________________________   _______________________________
Name of Practitioner (Please Print)   Name of Department (and specialty)

<u>Criteria for Granting of Privileges</u>:

One from each section is required with the supporting documentation attached.

_______ Completion of specialty/fellowship training that included a rotation in Anesthesia/Critical Care.

_______ Completion of training in a clinical subspecialty that provides training in Procedural Sedation.

_______ Completion of credentialing board requirements for advanced clinical practicum and completion of certification examination in Acute Care. **(Only for Nurse Practitioner)**

_______ Controlled Substance Prescriptive Authority Schedule II – V approval from the Mississippi Board of Nursing. **(Only for Nurse Practitioner)**

_______ Attendance/participation in an approved Procedural Sedation Training program.

_______ Provide a good-faith estimate of the number of instances of each type of procedure where sedation is administered with a list of any adverse events related to the sedation during those cases, including causal analysis, treatment, and outcome. This will demonstrate competence in the knowledge of agents including reversal agents, ability to manage cardiovascular instability and a compromised airway. **(Only for Physician and Dentist)**

_______ ACLS _______ PALS _______ NRP, as appropriate to patient population. **(Current)**

_______ Board Certification in Anesthesiology, Emergency Medicine, Interventional or Critical Care Specialties that include Procedural Sedation in the clinical training program.

_______ Other Board Certifications that include Procedural Sedation in the clinical training program and the use of vasoactive medications and airway management is done on a routine basis.

_______________________________ (specialty)

Statement of Applicant:
I have not requested privileges for any procedure for which I am not certified or eligible by training and experience for qualification. Furthermore, I realize that certification by a Board does not necessarily qualify me to perform certain procedures; however, I am competent to perform the procedure for which I have requested privileges.

_______________________________ _________ _______________________________ _________
Signature of Practitioner   **Date**   **Signature of Supervising Physician**   **Date**
    (If applicable)

I have reviewed and approve the above requested privileges and I attest that this practitioner is competent to perform the privileges requested.

_______________________________ _________
Signature of Department Chairman   **Date**

Revised 4/26/2005

FIG. 5-1

Example credentialing guidelines: Procedural sedation privileges and credentialing for staff physicians, dentists, residents, and nurse practitioners will require meeting one criterion from each section below. _(From the University of Mississippi Medical Center. Reprinted with permission.)_

    e. Reflux and aspiration risk
    f. Patient weight
2. **Caveat:** Ability to do 4 mets of exercise (e.g., walking four to five city blocks or going up two flights of stairs) is a very good predictor of adequate cardiopulmonary function.

C. Counsel the patient realistically about what to anticipate regarding:

1. Amnesia
2. Analgesia
3. Level of sedation
4. Side effects

D. By convention, the ASA classification is utilized to assess risk based on preexisting patient conditions.

1. ASA I: fit and healthy

**The University Hospitals and Clinics
Jackson, Mississippi**

Procedural Sedation Record

Addressograph

DATE: / /	TIME:	LOCATION:
Practitioner Performing Procedure:		PROCEDURE:
Practitioner Ordering Sedation:		☐ Arm Band in place and patient identity verified

Primary Language: ☐ English ☐ Spanish ☐ Other _________   Interpreter needed: ☐ No ☐ Yes, Name: _________

Transportation arranged with (name, relationship, phone): ☐ N/A

☐ Procedure & patient verified against signed consent form   ☐ N/A
☐ Side / Site verified   ☐ N/A   Weight: _________ lbs / _________ Kg   Age: _________

Belongings: ☐ Jewelry ☐Glasses ☐ Contacts ☐ Denture/Partials ☐ Hearing Aide   Disposition of Belongings:

Date/Time of last intake:

Adverse Reactions: (medications, food, latex) ☐ NKA

Current medications: ☐ None ☐ ASA ☐ Anticoagulant ☐ Cardiac Med ☐ NSAID ☐ Pain Med ☐ Herbals

List Other Med: ☐ See Attached

☐ Smoker ☐ Non-Smoker ☐ Alcohol Use ☐ Illicit Drug Use ☐ N/A

MEDICAL HISTORY	NO	YES	PHYSICAL ASSESSMENT - Practitioner	YES	NO	If "No", describe
Bleeding Disorder			NO Indication of difficult airway (See guidelines)			
Cancer			Ambulatory (age appropriate)			
Diabetes			Heart Rate Regular			
Dentures/Intra-oral devices			Neurological: Alert, age appropriate			
Snoring			Peripheral Pulses: Strong, equal			
Sleep Apnea			Lungs clear bilaterally			
Heart Disease			Teeth intact (not loose)			
Hypertension			Previous sedation: ☐ No ☐ Yes:			
Implantable Devices			Problems with previous anesthesia / sedation ☐ N/A ☐ No ☐ Yes:			
Kidney Disease			Aldrete score presedation: _________ (see guidelines)			
Liver Disease			COMMENTS:			
Lung Disease						
Pregnant						
Breast Feeding						
Seizures						
Stroke						
URI/Fever			Practitioner Signature:			

PROCEDURAL SEDATION PLAN / ORDERS: (Check those that apply)

1. IV: ☐ NS ☐ D5W ☐ _________   ☐ Saline Lock Rate: ☐ TKO or_________ ml/hr
2. Medication:
    ☐ Oxygen @ _________ LPM
    Titrate Med for Sedation (Circle route):
    ☐ Midazolam (Versed) _________ mg IV / PO   ☐ Nembutal _________ mg IV / IM / PO   ☐ Propofol _________ mg IV
    ☐ Fentanyl (Sublimaze) _________ mcg IV   ☐ Ketamine _________ mg IV / IM   ☐ Chloral hydrate _________ mg PO / PR
    ☐ Meperidine (Demerol) _________ mg IV   ☐ Methohexital (Brevital) _________ mg PR / IV   ☐ _________
    ☐ Morphine Sulfate _________ mg IV   ☐ Etomidate _________ mg IV
3. ☐ Prior to discharge, discontinue IV and provide discharge instructions
4. ☐ After procedure patient may be discharged when criteria met
    ☐ _________
    ☐ _________

Patient determined to be an appropriate candidate for sedation.   ASA Score (circle one): I   II   III IV E   (See Guidelines)
The risks, benefits, alternatives and resuscitation measures of the procedure and sedation have been explained to and understood by the patient/family. The attending MD of record agrees to proceed with procedural sedation.

Date/Time: _________

Practitioner Signature _________

Attending MD of record
☐ Present and agreed with findings as above
☐ Not present, discussed patient care and agreed

Catalog No. 1481 Revised 4/05   Page 1 of 4

FIG. 5-2

Example of a preprocedure evaluation form. *(From the University of Mississippi Medical Center. Reprinted with permission.)*   *(Continued)*

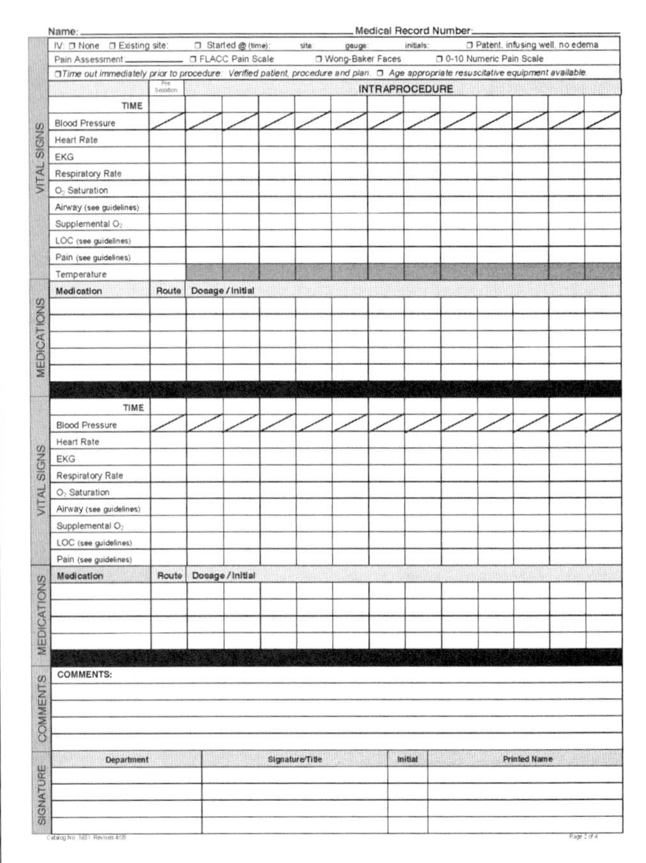

FIG. 5-2—cont'd

2. ASA II: mild systemic illness
3. ASA III: severe systemic illness that is not incapacitating
4. ASA IV: incapacitating, severe systemic illness
5. "E" is a modifier to indicate a nonelective procedure.

III. AIRWAY EVALUATION

A. Consists of four parts

1. Cervical range of motion: most important for C1–C2 extension. This may be estimated by the movement of the maxillary occlusal surface with extension (Fig. 5-3).

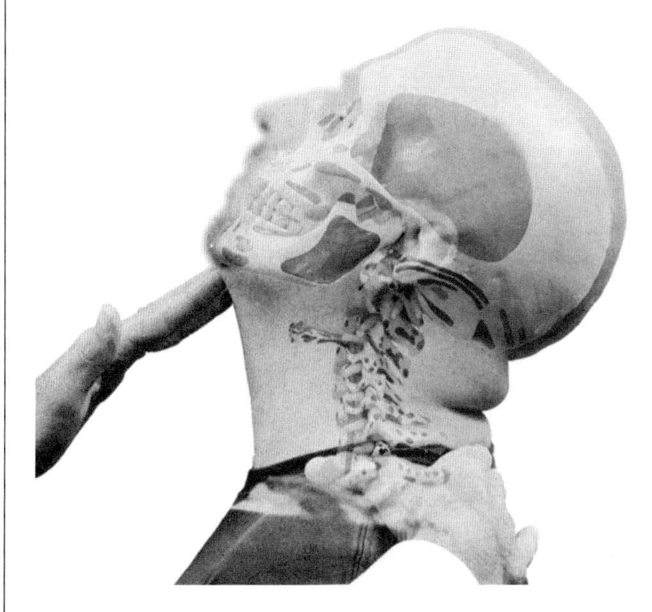

FIG. 5-3

Cervical range of motion must be at least 35 degrees.

2. Thyromental distance: distances form the upper thyroid cartilage to the posterior aspect of anterior mandible. Should be 2 to 3 fingerbreadths (3 to 4 cm if you have averaged-sized fingers) (Fig. 5-4).
3. Mandible excursion (mouth opening): should be at least 2 fingerbreadths or 4 cm (Fig. 5-5).
4. Posterior pharynx: you would like to see the tip of the uvula with the mouth open and tongue protruded. This estimates the amount of soft tissue that could impede your laryngoscopic view of the vocal cords (Fig. 5-6).
5. If you don't assess all four areas, you are again asking for trouble.

B. Things that predict a difficult airway:
1. History of a difficult airway
2. Obesity
3. Receding mandible
4. Protruding upper incisors
5. Loss of cervical mobility (extension) due to age or operations
6. Prior neck radiation therapy

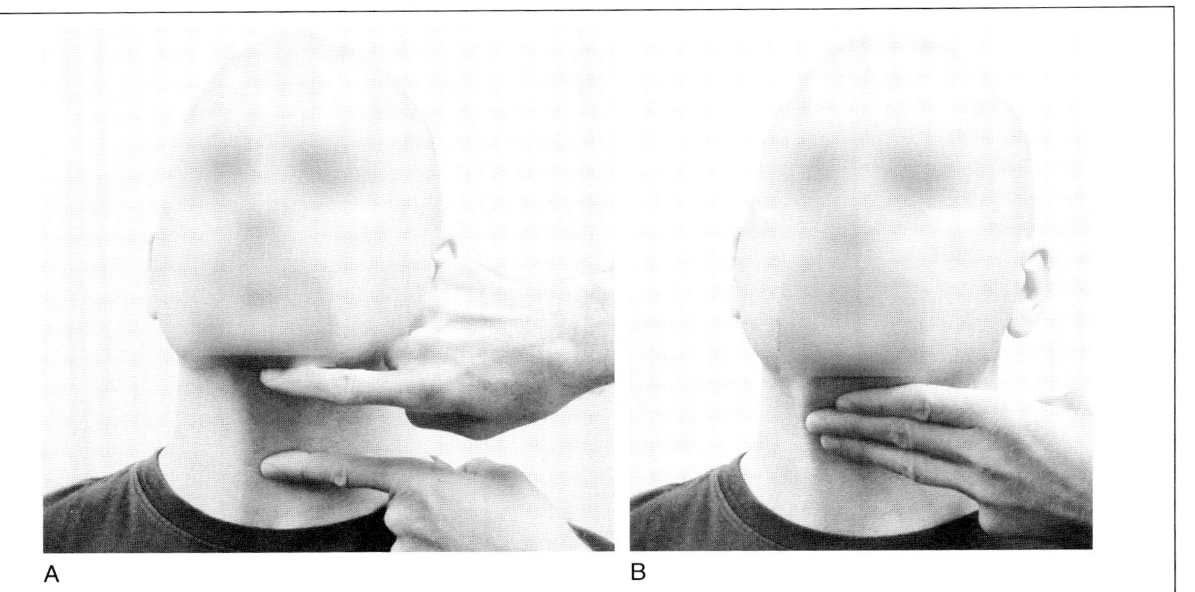

FIG. 5-4

Thyromental distance. A, Distance is measured between the upper border of the thyroid cartilage and the mentum (chin). B, Thyromental distance must be 2 to 3 fingerbreadths or more. If the distance is shorter, the larynx is considered anterior, and the Sellick maneuver (cricoid pressure) may be necessary to fully visualize the rima glottidis during direct laryngoscopy.

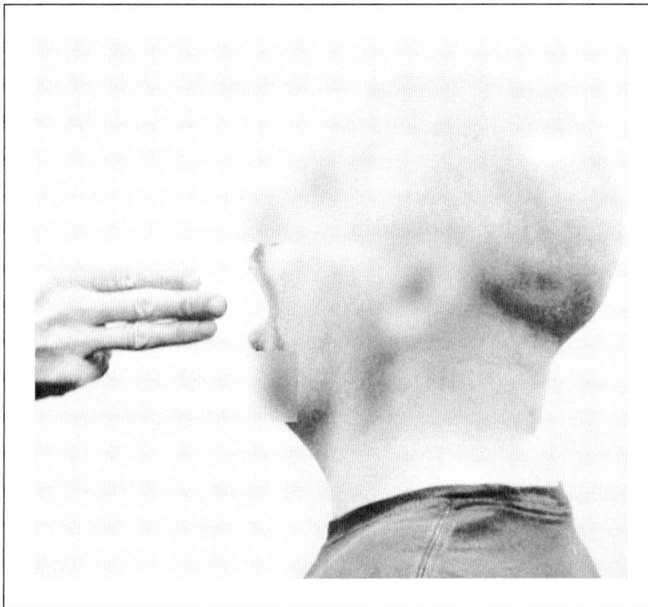

FIG. 5-5

Mouth opening. Mouth opening must be 2 to 3 fingerbreadths or more. Distance is likely increased after muscle relaxant is administered during induction.

C. Caveat: Do not sedate anyone you are not confident you can intubate; if you do, you are asking for trouble.

IV. EXAMPLE OF EQUIPMENT SET-UP

See Figure 5-7.

V. NPO GUIDELINES; RISK AND ASPIRATION PROPHYLAXIS

A. The risk for aspiration and the optimal duration of NPO are difficult to assess for procedural sedation practices.

B. Most good data and practice habits are directly linked to the general anesthesia literature.

C. With the exception of procedural sedation in the emergency department (where no one is ever NPO), it is advisable to adhere to the preprocedure ASA practice guidelines (Table 5-1).

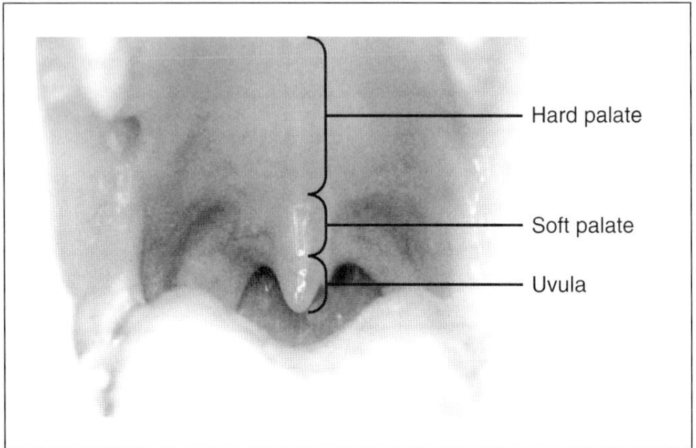

FIG. 5-6

Mallampati classification of pharyngeal view. Mallampati 1: full uvula is visible upon mouth opening with patient's tongue thrust out. Mallampati 2: uvula is partially visible. Mallampati 3: only soft palate is visible. Mallampati 4: only hard palate is visible.

D. Regarding pharmacologic manipulation of gastric volume and pH, no intervention is recommended for elective cases in which there is no obvious increased risk for pulmonary aspiration and the patient has been NPO.

E. For *emergency cases*, the proper duration of being NPO is poorly defined.
1. There is a risk for aspiration, but quantitation of this risk is extremely difficult.
2. The deeper the sedation, the more likely aspiration probably becomes.
3. You must make your own cautious clinical decisions.
4. Policy at our institution states: "Times should not be modified unless thoroughly documented that the procedure must be done on an emergency basis. If this patient experiences deep sedation, the patient must be intubated to protect the airway."

F. For *elective cases for patients at risk* (diabetes, states of altered gastric emptying, morbid obesity, hiatal hernia) consider metoclopramide, 10 to 20 mg IV, and an H_2 blocker (i.e., Pepcid, 20 to 40 mg IV) 30 to 60 minutes before anticipated start time.

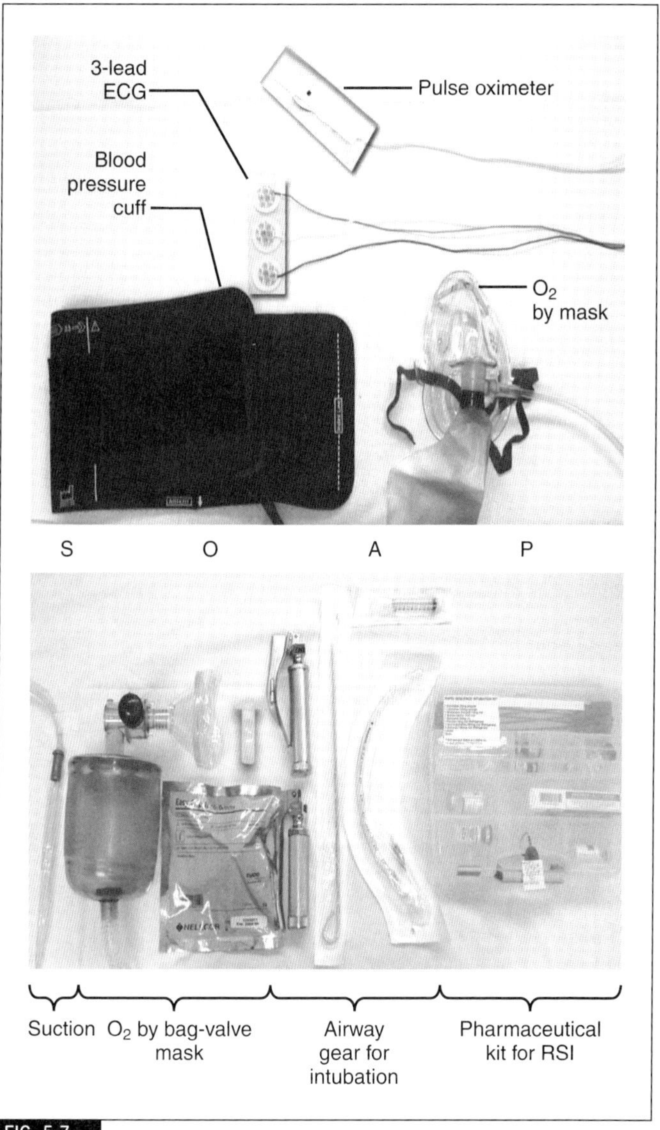

FIG. 5-7

Equipment setup for conscious sedation. *Top,* Standard monitors and O₂ supply. *Bottom,* Airway rescue setup. ECG, electrocardiogram; RSI, Rapid Sequence Induction.

TABLE 5-1

PREPROCEDURE AMERICAN SOCIETY OF ANESTHESIOLOGY
PRACTICE GUIDELINES

Ingested Material	Minimum Fasting Period
Clear liquids	2 hr
Breast milk	4 hr
Infant formula	6 hr
Nonhuman milk	6 hr
Light meal	6 hr

G. For *emergent and urgent cases*, such as fracture manipulation in the emergency department, consider nonparticulate antacid (sodium citrate [Bicitra], 30 mL) 5 to 10 minutes before starting. (Particulate antacids increase the severity of the aspiration pneumonitis.)

Note: *If aspiration or airway risk is deemed too high, consider "punting" the case to the operating room for a formal rapid-sequence induction by the anesthesia team.*

VI. MONITORING AND RECOVERY

A. Basic ASA monitors include:
1. Continuous three-lead electrocardiogram (ECG)
2. Blood pressure cuff
3. Pulse oximeter
4. Respiratory rate
5. Baseline temperature

B. Every 5 minutes (at a minimum):
1. Level of consciousness (LOC)
2. Heart rate and rhythm, blood pressure, respiratory rate
3. O_2 saturation
4. Airway patency
5. Pain reports

C. During recovery
1. Full baseline vital signs as noted above
2. Then *every* 15 minutes × 4
3. Then *every* 30 minutes × 2
4. Or until discharge criteria are met

D. If a patient receives a reversal agent (e.g., naloxone), the patient must be monitored an additional 90 minutes after the procedure.

E. Key components of discharge criteria include:
1. Level of consciousness and vital signs at presedation levels.

2. Patent airway
3. Pain score ≤ 4/10

F. Caveat: Look for preprocedure mental status, vital signs, and pain levels before discharge or transfers. Note absence of new issues such as nausea and vomiting or drug reactions.

BIBLIOGRAPHY

Practice guidelines for management of the difficult airway. *Anesthesiology* 1993; 78:597–602.
Practice guidelines for preoperative fasting and the use of pharmacologic agents to reduce the risk of pulmonary aspiration: Application to healthy patients undergoing elective procedures. *Anesthesiology* 1999; 90:896.
Practice guidelines for sedation and analgesia by non-anesthesiologists. *Anesthesiology* 1996; 84:447–459.
University of Mississippi Medical Center Procedural Sedation Policy. Procedural Sedation Committee. July 2005.

PROCEDURAL SEDATION **5**

Procedural Sedation Medication Choices

W. James Phillips, Christopher Decker, and Nathan Shefveland

I. BENZODIAZEPINES

Midazolam (Versed), diazepam (Valium), and lorazepam (Ativan)

A. History

Benzodiazepines produce five pharmacologic effects: sedation, anxiolysis, anterograde amnesia, muscle relaxation, and anticonvulsant actions. They facilitate action of the inhibitory neurotransmitter, γ-aminobutyric acid (GABA-A).

B. Usefulness

1. Primary use is as amnesic-sedative adjunct used to provide anxiolysis.
2. Sedation: preoperative and postoperative
3. Induction and maintenance of anesthesia
4. Indications
a. **U.S. Food and Drug Administration (FDA) approved:** sedation, anxiety, anesthesia, muscle relaxant, anticonvulsant
b. **Off label:** acute insomnia, irritable bowel syndrome, panic attack, depression, premenstrual syndrome, acute alcohol withdrawal syndrome
5. Procedural sedation utilization:
a. Most of the time, these agents are used as part of a combination technique in which benzodiazepines are administered to provide a "base" of anxiolysis and amnesia, after which a pure analgesic such as fentanyl is given or a pure sedative such as propofol for the more painful part of the procedure.
b. It is critical to understand that although the benzodiazepines may function as "solo" agents for procedural sedation, many practitioners believe that the doses required produce too much respiratory depression and too long-lasting an effect—even for midazolam.

C. Pharmacokinetics

See Table 6-1.

TABLE 6-1

PHARMACOKINETICS OF BENZODIAZEPINES

Drug (IV)	Onset	Duration	Protein Binding	Elimination Half-Life	Metabolism
Midazolam	1–5 min	15–60 min	95%	1–4 hr	Hepatic
Diazepam	<1 min	20–30 min	98%	20–50 hr	Hepatic
Lorazepam	5–20 min	4–8 hr	85%	12–16 hr	Hepatic

D. Routes and doses
See Table 6-2.

E. Formulations
1. Midazolam: 1 mg/mL, 5 mg/mL (injection solution); 2 mg/mL (syrup)
2. Diazepam: gel, rectal (Diastat); 5 mg/mL rectal tip (4.4 or 6 cm);
   5 mg/mL (injection solution); 5 mg/mL (oral solution); 2 mg, 5 mg,
   10 mg (tablet, Valium)
3. Lorazepam: 2 mg/mL (injection solution); 2 mg/mL (oral solution);
   0.5 mg, 1 mg, 2 mg (tablet)

F. Advantages
1. Reliable anterograde amnesia not provided by propofol, opiates, or
   barbiturates/etomidate
2. Midazolam is faster acting than diazepam and lorazepam.
3. Dose dependent effect (anxiolysis < amnesia < sedation)
4. Raises seizure threshold
5. Abruptly terminates seizures

G. Disadvantages
1. No analgesia
2. Hypotension
3. Respiratory depression that is ADDITIVE with other sedatives
4. Drug interactions: central nervous system (CNS) depressants, levodopa,
   loxapine, scopolamine, theophylline

H. Clinical pearls
1. Many practitioners feel that midazolam has rendered diazepam
   obsolete.
2. Midazolam is 2 or 3 times as potent as diazepam.
3. Beware of thrombophlebitis with diazepam, not seen with midazolam.

TABLE 6-2

ROUTES AND DOSES OF BENZODIAZEPINES

Drug	Adult Dose	Pediatric Dose
Midazolam	IV: 0.01–0.03 mg/kg	IV: 0.01 mg/kg min
	Cont. infusion: 25–50 mg/250 mL	Cont. infusion: same as adults
	D5W or NS—titrate; start at	IM: 0.1–0.15 mg/kg (max: 10 mg)
	0.01–0.03 mg/kg/hr	PO: 0.25–1 mg/kg
	IM: 0.07–0.08 mg/kg (usually	
	5 mg)	
Diazepam	IV, IM: 2–10 mg	IM, IV: 0.04–0.3 mg/kg
	PO: 2–10 mg	PO: 0.12–0.8 mg/kg
Lorazepam	IV, IM: 2 mg or 0.04 mg/kg	IV, IM, PO: 0.05–0.08 mg/kg
	Cont. infusion: 25 mg/250 mL	Cont. infusion: same as adults
	D5W or NS—titrate	
	PO: 1–4 mg	

4. Midazolam has a clinical dose-response curve:
a. 0.02–0.05 mg/kg = anxiolysis
b. 0.05–0.1 mg/kg = sedation, amnesia
c. 0.1–0.2 mg/kg = induction of anesthesia
5. Midazolam is a very common combination agent administered before fentanyl.
6. Midazolam is also commonly given before ketamine for procedural sedation to decrease emergence agitation and dysphoria.
7. Midazolam may also be administered IM, PO (as a pediatric premedication at 0.5 mg/kg), and intranasally as a pediatric premedication.

II. BARBITURATES

Pentobarbital (Nembutal), methohexital (Brevital), and thiopental (Pentothal)

A. History
Barbiturates are derived from barbituric acid. They produce sedative-hypnotic effects through the inhibitory neurotransmitter GABA-A in the CNS.

B. Usefulness
Sedation, induction, and maintenance of anesthesia, treatment of increased intracranial pressure (ICP)
1. Indications:
a. **FDA approved:** preanesthetic sedative, anticonvulsant
b. **Off label:** short-term treatment of insomnia
2. Procedural sedation indications:
a. Methohexital and thiopental are useful for deep sedation for BRIEF painful procedures.
b. Pentobarbital is useful as a PO sedative for pediatric cases that are not expected to be painful such as CT scan, etc.

C. Pharmacokinetics
See Table 6-3.

D. Routes and doses
See Table 6-4.

TABLE 6-3

PHARMACOKINETICS OF BARBITURATES

Drug (IV)	Onset	Duration	Protein Binding	Elimination Half-Life	Metabolism
Pentobarbital	<1 min	15 min	35%–55%	15–50 hr	Hepatic
Methohexital	10–20 sec	20–30 min	85%	3–5 hr	Hepatic
Thiopental	10–20 sec	20–30 min	85%–89%	8–10 hr	Hepatic

TABLE 6-4

ROUTES AND DOSES OF BARBITURATES

Drug	Adult Dose	Pediatric Dose
Pentobarbital	IV: 2–15 mg/kg IM: 150–200 mg	IV: 1–3 mg/kg PO, PR, IM: 3–5 mg/kg
Methohexital	IV: 1–1.5 mg/kg Cont. infusion: 30–100 µg/kg/min	IV: 1–1.5 mg/kg Cont. infusion: 1.9 mg/kg/min of 0.1% solution
Thiopental	IV: 2–4 mg/kg	IV: 2–3 mg/kg

E. Formulations

1. Pentobarbital: 50 mg/mL (injection solution)
2. Methohexital, thiopental: 500 mg, 2.5 g, 5 g (injection, powder for reconstitution)
3. Thiopental: 250 mg, 400 mg, 500 mg, 1 g, 2.5 g, 5 g (Pentothal)

F. Advantages

1. Dose-dependent amnesia
2. Dose-dependent drowsiness
3. Hypnosis
4. Drug of choice for elevated ICP

G. Disadvantages

1. Respiratory depression
2. Decreased systemic vascular resistance (SVR) = hypotension if volume depleted
3. No analgesia
4. Highly addictive with prolonged use
5. Adverse effects
a. Respiratory depression
b. Cardiovascular depression due to vasodilation
c. Myoclonus
d. Painful injection
e. Methohexital lowers seizure threshold, unlike other barbiturates.

H. Clinical pearls

1. Reliably produces hypotension.
2. Clinically useful IV doses of methohexital and thiopental will cause at least *some* respiratory depression.
3. Methohexital duration parallels that of propofol.
4. The effects, side effects, and recovery profile of methohexital and propofol are nearly identical.
5. Barbiturates are the drugs of choice for procedural sedation and airway management cases in which high ICP is suspected.

III. ETOMIDATE (AMIDATE)

A. History

Etomidate (Amidate, Hypnomidate), a short-acting nonbarbiturate hypnotic, was synthesized in the mid-1960s and first used in clinical practice in the early 1970s.

B. Usefulness

Induction of general anesthesia and brief procedural sedation in patients with cardiovascular disease, reactive airway disease, or **hemodynamic instability**

1. Indications:
a. **FDA approved:** induction of general anesthesia
b. **Off label:** procedural sedation of critically ill and ventilator-dependent patients
2. Procedural sedation indications:
a. Procedural sedation for brief painful procedures, as with barbiturates and propofol
b. Outstanding choice in cases of volume depletion or low cardiac reserve

C. Pharmacokinetics

See Table 6-5.

D. Routes and doses

1. Sedation: 0.2 to 0.3 mg/kg IV
Continuous infusion: 10 to 20 µg/kg per minute (rarely used, and safety concerns exist)

E. Formulations

Injection solution: 2 mg/mL (contains propylene glycol 35%)

F. Advantages

1. Rapid onset
2. Hemodynamic stability
3. Minimal effect on ventilation
4. Minimal effect on cardiovascular function
5. No histamine release
6. Raises seizure threshold

G. Disadvantages

1. Avoid use in pregnant and lactating females and children younger than 10 years. Prolonged sedation periods inhibit corticosteroid and

TABLE 6-5

PHARMACOKINETICS OF ETOMIDATE

Onset	Duration	Protein Binding	Elimination Half-Life	Metabolism
20 sec	4–10 min	76%	3 hr	Hepatic

mineralocorticoid synthesis, which is clinically significant with infusions. Infusions are not used clinically and might be considered contraindicated.

2. Adverse effects

a. Drug interactions: verapamil

b. Renal and hepatic function impairment

c. Nausea, vomiting, pain on injection, myoclonus, hiccups

H. Clinical pearls

1. Myoclonus seen in up to 20% of patients; do not confuse with seizure activity
2. Recovery time after single bolus dose 3 to 6 minutes, as with methohexital and propofol
3. Also lowers ICP, and so is another good choice in these cases, as with thiopental and propofol
4. Its true niche is for cases requiring sedation or intubation in the face of actual or potential hemodynamic instability.
5. For these patients, although the target dose is 0.2 to 0.3 mg/kg, consider titrating to this amount with 2-mg incremental doses every 15 seconds, in order to even more reliably avoid "overshoot" and hypotension.

IV. PROPOFOL (DIPRIVAN)

A. History

Propofol (Diprivan), an ultra-short-acting hypnotic, was developed in the 1970s and is the most frequently used IV anesthetic today. This alkyl phenol is commonly administered as an isotonic emulsion.

B. Usefulness

Induction and maintenance of sedation in adults. Induction of anesthesia in patients $\geq$ 3 years, and maintenance of anesthesia in patients > 2 months

1. Indications

a. **FDA approved:** sedation during diagnostic procedures; anesthesia induction and maintenance

b. **Off-label:** conscious sedation; postoperative antiemetic

2. Procedural sedation indications

a. As a bolus technique for brief painful procedures (adult = 1 mg/kg; children = 2 to 3 mg/kg)

b. In this regard, it may be considered interchangeable with etomidate and methohexital.

c. As an infusion for sedation for longer procedures at doses of 25 to 100 μg/kg per minute

C. Pharmacokinetics

See Table 6-6.

TABLE 6-6

PHARMACOKINETICS OF PROPOFOL (FOR BOLUS INJECTION OF 2.5 MG/KG)

Onset	Duration	Protein Binding	Elimination Half-Life	Metabolism
30 sec	3–5 min	97%–99%	3–12 hr	Hepatic

D. Routes and doses

1. Sedation (induction): IV infusion of 25 to 100 µg/kg per minute or bolus injection of 0.5 to 1.0 mg/kg (1 to 2 times higher in children)
2. Maintenance: IV infusion 25 to 100 µg/kg per minute or intermittent injection of 10 to 20 mg
3. "Poor man's infusion": Diprivan, titrated to desired end point

E. Formulations

1. Diprivan 1%: 10 mg/mL
2. Diprivan 2%: 20 mg/mL

F. Advantages

Rapid onset, quick recovery and return to consciousness, lower risk for nausea and vomiting

G. Disadvantages

1. Not recommended for pregnant or lactating females
2. Does not reliably provide amnesia
3. Adverse effects
a. Hypotension, bradycardia, headache, dystonic or choreiform movements, apnea, respiratory acidosis, hyperlipidemia or hypertriglyceridemia, painful injection, rash
b. Do not use in patients with a known allergy to egg or soybean protein.
c. With prolonged infusions, Diprivan may change respiratory quotient.

H. Clinical pearls

1. Propofol enjoys a hallowed place in the procedural sedation world owing to its immediate but brief duration and relative lack of a drug hangover.
2. This rapid metabolism allows the drug to also be delivered by an infusion.
3. It is an intense sedative that provides minimal if any amnesia and questionable analgesia.
4. Caution must still be exercised owing to its ability to cause respiratory depression and hypotension, especially in elderly patients.
5. Mix with lidocaine to decrease pain on injection (10 mg lidocaine/10 mL Diprivan).
6. Use caution in elderly patients; consider alternatives if age > 65 years.
7. Apnea is reliably produced with bolus dosing.

V. OPIOIDS FOR SEDATION

A. Fentanyl (Sublimaze)

1. Overview

Fentanyl citrate is a potent, highly lipid-soluble synthetic opioid of the phenylpiperidine group that is useful for short-term analgesia and sedation most commonly in the perioperative setting or during procedural sedation.

2. Indications and usage

a. Because of its lipid solubility, fentanyl has a rapid onset of action of 3 to 5 minutes and a **duration of analgesic action of 30 minutes.** It is then redistributed from the CNS into tissues with an elimination half-life of 3 hours.

b. A dose of 100 µg (0.1 mg; 2.0 mL) is about equivalent in analgesic activity to 10 mg or morphine or 75 mg of meperidine.

c. Starting doses of fentanyl for procedural sedation should be **1–2 µg/kg,** titrated every 3 to 5 minutes in **0.25 to 0.5 µg/kg** increments until adequate sedation is achieved.

3. **Metabolism:** primarily transformed in the liver to inactive metabolites

4. **Advantages**

a. Rapid onset of action compared to morphine

b. Short half-life

c. Produces **less histamine release** than morphine-like opioids and thus has fewer cardiovascular effects and less hypotension

d. Potentially less emetic activity than morphine or meperidine

5. Disadvantages

a. Short duration of action, may require more frequent dosing.

b. Respiratory depression may last longer than analgesia.

6. Clinical pearls

a. Fentanyl may be preferred to morphine for the relief of pain in patients who may be **volume depleted or are dependent on cardiac preload** (the "etomidate" of opioids).

b. Fentanyl is most often utilized as a combination technique with a benzodiazepine such as midazolam.

c. Remember that opioids are basically just analgesics, with no amnesia potential and clinical sedation occurring only at higher doses; hence the need for these agents to typically be used in combination with other drugs that will more reliably provide true sedation and amnesia.

B. Alfentanil (Alfenta), sufentanil (Sufenta), and remifentanil

1. Overview

Remifentanil, alfentanil, and sufentanil are also potent, highly lipid-soluble synthetic opioids of the phenylpiperidine group. Their main advantage compared with fentanyl are shorter durations of action. Comparisons to fentanyl are as follows (drug dose half-life):

a. Fentanyl: 1 to 5 µg/kg ± 30 minutes

b. Sufentanil: 0.1 to 0.5 µg/kg ± 15 minutes

c. Alfentanil: 5 to 20 µg/kg ± 10 minutes

d. Remifentanil: 0.5 to 1 µg/kg minutes
2. Clinical pearls
a. Remifentanil is rapidly metabolized by nonspecific plasma esterases, and its effects are extraordinarily brief.
b. The use of remifentanil and, to a degree, alfentanil, for procedural sedation would be for EXTREMELY BRIEF procedures unless the drug was given as an infusion. In this sense, the applicability of these agents would be the same as for single-dose sedatives such as propofol, etomidate, and methohexital for brief painful procedures.
c. To use these rapidly acting agents successfully, it is essential to have the person reducing the dislocation or manipulating the fracture poised and ready to start as the medication begins to be titrated. This ensures that the procedure can be started as soon as the peak analgesia is achieved.
d. PRECAUTION: These highly potent opioids may exhibit profound respiratory depression and *chest wall rigidity* when larger doses are given *and* with rapid bolus techniques. This may be so profound as to inhibit ventilation and require intravenous paralytics.

VI. KETAMINE (KETALAR)

A. Overview

Ketamine is treated separately because of its unique properties and differences from other nonopioid intravenous anesthetics. It is a highly lipid-soluble agent packaged as a racemic mixture of the S(+) and R(−) enantiomers. The S(+) enantiomer is responsible for most of the analgesic activity, whereas the R(−) may cause most of the psychomimetic phenomena.

B. Usefulness

1. Ketamine is unique in that it is a sedative, amnestic, and *intense analgesic*. The analgesic effect is due to a dissociation between the cortex and thalamic and limbic systems (dissociative anesthesia). With variances in doses, ketamine may be used for analgesia, procedural sedation, and induction and maintenance of general anesthesia (Table 6-7).
2. Procedural sedation utilization

TABLE 6-7

USES OF KETAMINE

Use	IV Dose	IM Dose
Analgesia	0.15–0.25 mg/kg	
Procedural sedation	0.25–1 mg/kg	2–4 mg/kg
Induction of general anesthesia	2 mg/kg	4–6 mg/kg
Maintenance of general anesthesia	30–90 µg/kg/min	

a. As with all parenteral sedatives, careful titration is the key. With a 30- to 60-second onset time, target effects may be seen quickly.
b. Although ketamine is amnestic, presedation administration of midazolam 0.01 to 0.03 mg/kg will decrease the incidence of **emergence delirium** from ketamine.
c. Target ketamine IV dose ranges for sedation = 0.25 to 1 mg/kg. A technique is to titrate 10 to 30 mg at a time with 30 to 60 seconds between each dose.
d. This will generally provide analgesia for 15 to 25 minutes.
e. Ketamine may be mixed with propofol, allowing about half of the usual sedative dose for both. (Example: 10 mL syringe = 50 mg propofol, 50 mg ketamine = 5 mg/mL of both agents)
f. Ketamine may also be given orally in a dose range of 5 to 10 mg/kg with onset time of 30 to 45 minutes and duration of 30 to 45 minutes.
g. Because of the intense analgesia provided, supplemental opioids are rarely needed.
h. **Emergence delirium** can be a true problem. Attempt to awaken the patient in a calm, quiet, and darkened environment.

C. Pharmacokinetics
1. Clinical onset after IV use = 30 seconds to 1 minute
2. Distribution half-life = 12 to 16 minutes
3. Clinical recovery time after bolus dose = 15 to 30 minutes
4. Higher doses produce prolonged recovery times.
5. Metabolism
a. Metabolized by hepatic microsomal enzymes.
b. Major pathway yields nor-ketamine, an active metabolite with some renal excretion.

D. Routes and doses
Although used primarily IV and IM, ketamine has also been administered orally, rectally, nasally, and when available as a preservative free solution, epidurally. Its action at the spinal cord may be due to:
1. Na^+ and Ca^{++} channel modulation
2. Agonism at spinal opiate receptors
3. Agonism at spinal sigma receptors
4. *N*-methyl-D-aspartate (NMDA) receptor antagonism (present in CNS and peripheral nervous system; this also explains the ability of ketamine to block or delay opiate tolerance and to exert an analgesic effect in cases of opiate resistant chronic or neuropathic pain)

E. Formulations
1. 1%, 5%, and 10% solutions—racemic mixtures
2. S(+) enantiomer as now available as a 0.5% and 2.5% concentration (5 mg/mL and 25 mg/mL).

F. Organ system effects
1. CNS
a. Increase cerebral blood flow (CBF).
b. Patients appear cataleptic.
c. **Usually** preserves airway reflexes, open eyes, mild papillary dilation, ± nystagmus, increased lacrimation, and salivation
2. Cardiovascular system
a. Elevated heart rate and blood pressure through sympathetic nervous system activation (**usually** overshadows its direct myocardial depressant action)
b. Increased work, myocardial O_2 consumption
3. Pulmonary
a. Usually maintains a stable respiratory rate and depth
b. Rare apnea or loss of airway reflex
c. Bronchial smooth muscle relaxant
d. Elevation of pulmonary vascular resistance

VII. NITROUS OXIDE (N_2O)

A. Overview
1. Nitrous oxide is an odorless and colorless sedative and analgesic gas that is the only inorganic anesthetic gas in clinical use. It is manufactured by heating ammonium nitrate and compressed for use in tanks as a liquid. The liquid rapidly equilibrates with its gaseous phase, so that tanks of N_2O contain both, with the gas being inhaled by the patient. Clinically useful concentrations are 40% to 70%.
2. N_2O is nonexplosive and nonflammable but may support combustion equally as well as oxygen.
3. N_2O is highly soluble (35 times more soluble than nitrogen) and once inhaled, travels rapidly from the lungs into the bloodstream and to the vessel-rich organs.
4. The mechanism of action of N_2O in the CNS is speculative, with probabilities including cellular membrane deformities and CNS opioid receptor stimulation.
5. The onset of action after inhalation is 2 to 3 minutes with a similar "off gas" time to recovery after discontinuation. N_2O undergoes minimal, if any, biotransformation and is exhaled unchanged without production of metabolites or organ toxicity.
6. N_2O is a teratogen, so frequent or continuous use should be avoided in pregnant patients and in pregnant health care professionals with clinical exposure. N_2O may also cause bone marrow depression, so scavenging systems should be in place in areas of use.

B. Organ system effects of N_2O include the following:
1. *CNS*: Mild increase in cerebral blood flow and ICP
2. *Cardiovascular*: Like ketamine, N_2O is an in vitro direct cardiac depressant but a sympathetic nervous system activator. Unless the patient is hypovolemic or in severe shock or stress, the latter effect is

seen clinically with a modest rise in heart rate and blood pressure. However, an increase in both systemic and pulmonary vascular resistance is seen.

3. *Respiratory*: Although N_2O causes a rise in respiratory rate, a dip in tidal volume results in a modest decrease in minute ventilation. Of particular note is the marked depression of carotid body sensitivity to arterial hypoxemia.
4. *Renal and hepatic*: Modest decreases in blood flow to both systems is observed.
5. *GI*: An increased incidence in nausea and vomiting is likely mediated through stimulation of the CNS chemoreceptor trigger zone.

C. Contraindications
1. Severe shock
2. Hypoxia requiring higher concentrations of oxygen
3. Pulmonary hypertension
4. State where sympathetic stimulation would be extremely detrimental (coronary ischemia, insufficiency)
5. The presence of trapped air
a. Pneumocephalus
b. Pneumothorax
c. Intraocular air
d. Small bowel obstruction
e. **The high diffusibilty of N_2O would cause it to diffuse into and EXPAND these areas.**

D. Procedural sedation utilization
1. N_2O should be delivered through a two-tank system with oxygen and include a linkage and mixing valve that ensures a lower limit of fraction of inspired O_2 (FiO_2) (typically 0.3) and cuts off the N_2O if the oxygen supply fails or runs out.
2. Full patient monitoring is required, with end-tidal CO_2 ($ETCO_2$) desirable.
3. Clinically useful concentrations are usually 50% to 70% in oxygen, with the higher ranges producing more sedation.
4. Patients will become more sedated (but often not asleep) after inhaling N_2O for 1 to 3 minutes. Waking time after discontinuation is about the same.
5. Consider N_2O a moderate sedative and analgesic providing adequate conditions for minor procedures such as:
a. Difficult IV access
b. Central line placement
c. Dental work
d. Laceration repair
e. Minor facture manipulation
f. Very uncomplicated single-move joint reductions
6. At conclusion of the procedure, patients should receive 100% O_2 for several minutes to minimize diffusion hypoxia.

7. For more complicated or painful procedures, N_2O may be used as a combination agent.

a. Procedures in which sedation-**amnesia** is more critical than dense analgesia: base of IV sedative such as midazolam, 0.03 to 0.05 mg/kg, followed in 3 to 5 minutes by N_2O inhalation, 50% to 70%.

b. Procedures in which analgesia is more critical or the procedure is anticipated to be extremely painful:

   (1) Base of IV analgesic such as fentanyl, 1 to 4 µg/kg, or morphine, 0.08 to 0.15 mg/kg

   (2) Followed in 3 to 5 minutes by inhalation of 50% to 70% N_2O.

E. Caveats for N_2O use:

1. Fast on/fast off with minimal residual effect. There is no lasting sedation *or* analgesia. Patients may require parenteral analgesics for residual postprocedure pain.
2. Excellent agent for minor to modestly stimulating procedures. Need to use in combination with parenteral agents for extremely painful or stimulating events.
3. Respiratory and sedative effects from N_2O are *additive* with parenteral sedatives and analgesics.
4. Beware the potential for HYPOXIA because N_2O is diluting the delivered O_2 concentration. Meticulous attention to airway adequacy, ventilation, and oxygen saturation is critical.
5. Beware the potential for cardiorespiratory depression in the critically ill, injured, hypovolemic, elderly, or chronically ill.

VIII. PUTTING THE PIECES TOGETHER

Sedation techniques vary widely, and any agent may be used in a variety of circumstances.

A. For brief painful procedures such as joint or fracture manipulation and cardioversions; consider a *bolus sedative* technique:

1. Propofol: 1 to 1.5 mg/kg/IV or
2. Methohexital: 0.5 to 1 mg/kg/IV or
3. Etomidate: 0.2 to 0.3 mg/kg/IV
4. Advantages:
a. Brief "dense" sedation and muscle relaxation
b. Rapid recovery
5. Disadvantages
a. Potential respiratory depression
b. Hypotension (less likely with etomidate)
c. **Pain** if inadequately dosed
6. Caveat: Although these agents are sedatives with no intrinsic analgesic action, at induction-level doses, the clinical effect appears to be sedation and analgesia. The CNS is "put to sleep."

B. For *longer*, more painful procedures, such as complex laceration repairs, consider:

1. Midazolam, 0.01 to 0.03 mg/kg, followed by ketamine, 1 to 1.5 mg/kg
a. Midazolam reinforces amnesia and decreases emergence delirium.
b. Ketamine effect lasts 15 to 30 minutes and may be redosed.

OR

2. Midazolam, 0.01 to 0.03 mg/kg IV, followed by fentanyl, 2 to 4 µg/kg, or morphine, 0.1 to 0.15 mg/kg IV
a. Midazolam provides amnesia-sedation.
b. Morphine or fentanyl provides 30 to 45 minutes of modest analgesia.

OR

3. Midazolam, 0.01 to 0.02 mg/kg IV, followed by inhalation of 50% to 70% N_2O by face mask. Remember, N_2O provides no residual analgesia.
4. Caveat: Beware additive respiratory depression with ALL these and any combination sedative-analgesic technique.

C. For sedation or anxiolysis for nonpainful procedures, consider:

1. Lorazepam, 0.01 to 0.03 mg/kg PO or
2. Midazolam, 0.4 to 0.5 mg/kg PO or
3. Midazolam, 0.01 to 0.03 mg/kg IV titrated to sedation or
4. Propofol infusion (low dose), 10 to 25 µg/kg per minute

D. Infusion techniques

1. Almost any agent can be given as an infusion. The problem is that drug accumulation occurs and waking times may be greatly prolonged. There is also some danger from drug overdose, and meticulous attention is required during administration of sedation.
2. Realistically, the only agents discussed here that are amenable to infusion techniques for procedural sedation are the shorter-acting phenylpiperidines (e.g., remifentanil, alfentanil) and propofol. Ketamine infusions are well described for analgesia and sedation techniques, but their description is beyond the scope of this section. Using phenylpiperidine infusions should necessitate having the anesthesia team present.
3. Propofol, although not without its own potential respiratory depression and hypotension profile, may be more user friendly.
4. The three keys to using propofol infusions are:
a. A **syringe infusion pump** for dose ranges of 25 to 100 µg/kg per minute (yes, there are cowboys and cowgirls that just use a Mini drip IV set, but this can hardly be considered optimal)
b. A dedicated and trained **sedation specialist** (anesthesia personnel or RN) who is watching the patient like a hawk
c. Recognition that propofol infusions (as opposed to high dose single bolus therapy) provide **minimal clinical analgesia** and that short-acting opiates may be required during and after the procedure for pain

Pediatric Considerations

W. James Phillips and Loretta Jackson Williams

A. Overview
1. Although we use the same agents for adult and pediatric pain management, there are different and additional considerations in the pediatric population.
2. These differences include respiratory mechanics, drug metabolism, drug toxicity profiles, and airway anatomy should respiratory depression requiring airway rescue occur.
3. Young children have a relatively high oxygen consumption and lower functional residual volume with respect to weight. Desaturation occurs more quickly in the apneic patient. Airway obstruction also occurs more readily owing to the relatively larger tongue size in children. The larger pediatric occiput also forces the neck into flexion, requiring special attention to head positioning for airway management.
4. Infants and younger children have relatively immature hepatic enzyme systems, protein-binding capacity, and renal filtration parameters. Infants also have immature reflex responses to hypoxia and hypercarbia.
5. Although rates of maturation vary, most systems have matured by 6 to 9 months of age. Neonates and infants have relatively lower levels of α acid glycoprotein and albumin, which results in larger pharmacologically active fractions of drugs.
6. For children younger than 6 months, starting opiate doses should be reduced by 50% to 75% and then titrated as indicated.

B. Pain assessment in children:
1. A complete discussion of this complicated subject reaches far beyond the scope of this section. Do remember that children as young as the age of 2 years can provide some degree of verbal information about their pain.
2. Individual institutions should decide which scale to use for which age groups after input from a multidisciplinary pain management team.
3. Some common pain assessment tools include:
a. Visual analog scale: generally for school-aged children.
b. Oucher scale: combines a numerical scale with a series of photographs.
c. Colored analog scale: colors are assigned to varying degrees of pain.
d. Faces pain scale: six cartoon faces are shown that range from no pain to very much pain.
e. Body outline tool: the child draws an X on or colors in the area of pain.
f. Poker chips tool: the more chips, the more pain.

4. For nonverbal patients, more complex assessment tools that rely on behavior and physiologic clues are used. These may include:
a. Postoperative pain score (POPS)
b. Toddler-preschool POPS
c. Neonatal facial coding system
5. There are separate scales for procedural pain and for children with decreased cognitive abilities.

C. Nonsteroidal anti-inflammatory drugs

1. Nonsteroidal anti-inflammatory drugs (NSAIDs) agents inhibit cyclooxygenase (COX) enzyme systems, thereby lowering prostaglandin levels. COX enzyme systems convert arachidonic acid to different prostaglandins that may sensitize nociceptors, increase regional blood flow and inflammation, facilitate pain transmission, modulate regional blood flow (kidney), and protect the gastric mucosa.
2. NSAID clearance is reduced in neonates and infants, is increased relative to adults in children ages 3 to 8 years, and normalizes to adult levels by about age 10 years.
3. Two isoenzymes, COX-1 and COX-2, exist. The former is a constitutive enzyme that is present in many tissue beds in a steady state and serves to maintain protective levels of prostaglandins (i.e., gastric mucosa). The COX-2 isoenzyme is largely an inducible enzyme; that is, levels are increased in times of pain and inflammation.
4. Traditional COX inhibitors (older NSAIDs) are nonselective in that they likely inhibit both isoenzymes in a nonselective fashion. Therefore, although they provide good analgesia, they may also cause prostaglandin changes that are detrimental (gastric ulcer formation, renal insufficiency).
5. Some traditional COX-1 inhibitors have been termed *gastric-sparing NSAIDs*. These may include salsalate, diflunisal, choline magnesium salicylate (Trilisate), or nabumetone (Relafen, a prodrug later converted to active form). This terminology is not entirely accurate; although gastrointestinal (GI) side effects appear to be decreased, this may simply reflect lower prostaglandin inhibition and potentially less analgesic effect.
6. COX-2 inhibitors preferentially, *but not completely*, inhibit COX-2 enzymes, the more inducible enzymes of the COX system. This potentially avoids some of the traditional NSAID side effects. In reality, the main benefit for the COX-2 agents has been gastric protection. There does not appear to be significant renal protection as compared with the traditional agents.
7. The COX-2 isoenzyme is an inducible enzyme expressed predominantly in leukocytes and in neurons of the central and peripheral nervous systems. COX-2 inhibitors likely exert their effect through both a central and peripheral effort.

8. Regarding NSAID potency, there are *no* strong data to suggest that:
a. Newer NSAIDs are better than older ones.
b. COX-2 inhibitors are superior to COX-1.
c. Ketorolac is stronger than other NSAIDs; it probably just works faster.
9. NSAID advantages include:
a. Opiate sparing
b. No respiratory depression
c. No tolerance
d. No nausea or vomiting
10. NSAID disadvantages
a. Nephropathy
b. Gastropathy
c. Bleeding due to platelet inhibition (lower risk than in adults)
d. Exacerbation of hypertension
e. **NSAIDS may impair bone healing. Beware in patients at risk for fracture nonunion.**
11. COX-2 caveats:
a. Lower incidence of gastropathy
b. Perhaps less platelet inhibitor effect
c. No decrease in renal toxicity compared with nonselective agents
d. Rofecoxib and valdecoxib were withdrawn from the market because of cardiovascular toxicities in adults. Many of these cases were after prolonged (>6 months) utilization.
12. Acetaminophen
a. Minimal peripheral anti-inflammatory effects
b. Largely a central analgesic
c. Beware of different elixir strengths
d. Dosing
    (1) Starting dose: 10 to 20 mg/kg PO
    (2) Maximum daily dose
        (a) Children: 100 mg/kg
        (b) Term infants: 75 mg/kg
        (c) Premature infants: 40 mg/kg
    (3) Rectal dose: 30 to 45 mg/kg, then 20 mg/kg every 6 hours.
13. Ketorolac
a. Only parenteral NSAID
b. No stronger than other NSAIDs
c. May be given IV or IM
d. Has reported instances of bronchospasm, delayed bone healing, and postoperative bleeding
e. May be particularly effective in cases of renal colic and bladder spasms. Bladder prostaglandin levels are lowered.
f. Generally limit use to < 3 days
14. NSAID dosing guidelines (Table 7-1)

TABLE 7-1

NSAID DOSING GUIDELINES

	Weight < 60 kg	Weight > 60 kg
Acetaminophen	10–15 mg/kg every 4 hr PO	650–1000 mg every 4 hr PO
Naprosyn	5 mg/kg every 12 hr PO	250–500 mg every 12 hr PO
Ibuprofen	6–10 mg/kg every 6–8 hr PO	400–600 mg every 6–8 hr PO
Celebrex	2–4 mg/kg every 12 hr PO	100–200 mg every 12 hr PO
Ketorolac	0.5 mg/kg every 6–8 hr IV	30 mg every 6–8 hr IV

D. Opiates
1. The younger the child, the greater the risk for respiratory depression and prolonged opiate effect.
2. For children younger than 4 to 6 months, lower standard doses by 50% to 75%.
a. Example: morphine half-life in adults = 2 to 3 hours; morphine half-life in premature infants = 10 hours
3. Specific agent caveats
a. Codeine
   (1) Weak analgesic
   (2) Is only an analgesic because some gets converted to morphine
   (3) Some patients are poor converters and get minimal analgesia
   (4) Has a clinical ceiling effect—about 1.5 to 2 mg/kg; side effects may be intolerable
   (5) Usually combined with acetaminophen
b. Oxycodone
   (1) Available as an elixir or sustained tablet
   (2) Useful for severe pain
   (3) Comes singly or in combination with acetaminophen
   (4) Typical doses are 0.1 to 0.2 mg/kg every 4 hours.
c. Hydrocodone
   (1) Less potent than oxycodone
   (2) Available as an elixir
d. Morphine
   (1) First choice as pediatric parenteral opiate
   (2) May cause erythema and hives along the course of the vein—not an allergy
   (3) Decreases blood pressure by decreased systemic vascular resistance (SVR), pain relief, and vasodilation
   (4) Clinical half-life is about 2 to 3 hours
   (5) Undergoes hepatic conversion to 6 and 3 glucuronide—these contribute strongly to analgesia
   (6) Accumulates in renal failure
e. Hydromorphone
   (1) Hydrogenated ketone of morphine
   (2) 7 to 10 times more potent than morphine

       (3) Minimal accumulation in renal failure

       (4) Much more lipid soluble than morphine; more rapid onset and more euphoria

       (5) Useful substitute in cases of true morphine allergy

  f. Meperidine

       (1) Is a terrible drug—see Chapter 2, p. 10

       (2) You can certainly find a better substitute for this agent.

  g. Fentanyl

       (1) 70 to 100 times more potent than morphine

       (2) Minimal renal accumulation

       (3) Excellent hemodynamic stability

       (4) Repeated doses or infusions increase the clinical half-life.

       (5) Available as a transdermal preparation: 18 to 24 hours are needed to achieve steady state.

          (a) 25 = 25 μg/hour steady state

          (b) 50 = 50 μg/hour steady state

          (c) 75 = 75 μg/hour steady state

          (d) 100 = 100 μg/hour steady state

          (e) Each patch lasts 3 days.

  h. Methadone

       (1) Long acting

       (2) Variable half-life early on

       (3) *N*-methyl-D-aspartate (NMDA) blocker in addition to being a μ agonist

          (a) Dextro enantiomer = μ agonist

          (b) Levo enantiomer= NMDA receptor blocker

       (4) Available as an elixir

       (5) High bioavailability after oral use

       (6) 1 mg methadone = 3 mg morphine (arguable; older literature rates this as 1:1)

       (7) Methadone may be drug of choice in opiate-tolerant patients (incomplete cross-tolerance)

  i. Tramadol

       (1) Synthetic analogue of codeine

       (2) μ Agonism

       (3) Serotonin and norepinephrine reuptake blocker

       (4) Mechanisms of both opiates and tricyclics

       (5) Minimal sedation and respiratory depressions

       (6) Available: PO in United States; IV in Europe

       (7) Analgesia reversed by ondansetron (5-HT$_3$ blockage)

       (8) Mild analgesic

  j. Dextromethorphan

       (1) Popular antitussive

       (2) NMDA receptor blocker

       (3) Opiate sparing in postoperative pain studies

4. Pediatric analgesics available as elixirs (Table 7-2)

TABLE 7-2

PEDIATRIC ANALGESICS AVAILABLE AS ELIXIRS

Agent	Strength
Acetaminophen	Liquid: 160 mg/5 mL, 500 mg/15 mL
	Drops: 80 mg/0.8 mL
Ibuprofen	Liquid: 100 mg/5 mL, 100 mg/2.5 mL
	Drops: 50 mg/1.25 mL = infant drops in dropper
Oxycodone	5 mg/5 mL, concentrate 20 mg/mL
Hydrocodone	7.5/500 mg hydrocodone/acetaminophen/15 mL
(as Lortab Elixir)	
Codeine	15 mg/5mL
Morphine	10 mg/5 mL, 10 mg/2.5 mL, 20 mg/5 mL, 20 mg/mL
Methadone	5 and 10 mg/5mL
Hydromorphone	5 mg/mL

5. Opiate dosing guidelines for children = 6 months of age
a. For children < 50 kg (Table 7-3)
b. Opiate infusions for children 2 to 6 months of age
   (1) Morphine: 0.03 mg/kg per hour
   (2) Hydromorphone: 0.006 mg/kg per hour
   (3) Fentanyl: 0.5 to 2 µg/kg per hour
6. Opiate caveats
a. For opiate-induced itching:
   (1) Nalbuphine: 0.25 to 0.5 mg/kg IV every 6 hours
   (2) Naloxone infusion: 0.1 to 0.3 µg/kg per hour
      (a) Mix 10 µg/mL 0.9 NaCl
      (b) Also useful for refractory nausea
   (3) Hydroxyzine: 0.5 to 1.0 mg/kg PO every 6 hours
b. Nausea and vomiting
   (1) Metoclopramide: 0.05 to 0.15 mg/kg PO/IV every 8 hours
   (2) Ondansetron: 0.1 to 0.2 mg/kg IV every 8 hours (if >40 kg, 4 to 8 mg PO/IV)
   (3) Promethazine: 0.1 to 0.25 mg/kg PO every 6 hours

E. Pediatric intravenous patient-controlled analgesia (PCA):
1. Provides very stable blood levels.
2. Morphine is the most commonly used agent.
3. Lockout interval is usually 8 to 10 minutes.
4. Each dose must be individualized. Consider starting dose of 10 to 20 µg/kg (0.01 to 0.02 mg/kg).
5. Protocols may include background infusion.
6. Successfully used as young as age 5 years.
7. Carefully assess maturity, parental understanding, and parental support.
8. Nurse-controlled PCA is an efficient and time-saving technique. Vigilance is paramount to avoid oversedation.

TABLE 7-3

OPIATE DOSING GUIDELINES FOR CHILDREN 6 MONTHS OR OLDER AND WEIGHING LESS THAN 50 KG

Agent	Comparative Parenteral Doses	PO Dose	Starting IV Dose	Starting PO Dose
Codeine	120 mg	200 mg	Do not give IV	0.2–0.5 mg/kg every 4 hr
Hydrocodone	NA	30 mg	NA	0.05–0.1 mg/kg every 4–6 hr
Oxycodone	NA	10 mg	NA	0.1–0.2 mg/kg every 4–6 hr
Morphine	10 mg	30 mg	0.1 mg/kg every 2–3 hr	0.3 mg/kg every 3–4 hr
Methadone	3–5 mg	10 mg	0.05–0.1 mg/kg every 6–8 hr	0.1–0.2 mg/kg every 6–8 hr
Hydromorphone	2 mg	4 mg	0.015 mg/kg every 2–4 hr	0.04–0.06 mg/kg every 3–4 hr
Fentanyl	100 μg	NA	0.5–2.0 μg/kg every 1–2 hr	NA
Meperidine	100 mg	300 mg	0.25–1 mg/kg every 3 hr	2–3 mg/kg every 4 hr

9. Hydromorphone is considered an excellent second-line agent if morphine is not appropriate. Remember hydromorphone dose DOES NOT EQUAL morphine dose.
10. Maintain a low threshold for using continuous pulse oximetry in higher-risk cases.

II. PROCEDURAL SEDATION CONSIDERATIONS

A. Background

There are a number of painful noninvasive and invasive procedures performed for children outside of the traditional operating room setting. In addition, the public's expectation for protection from pain during medical treatment is high. Part of this expectation is supported by the knowledge that individuals of all ages experience pain. Despite that knowledge, there is evidence that infants and children receive less analgesia than adults for comparable procedures. This chapter provides some guidelines for appropriate use of sedation in the pediatric population and reviews the pharmacology of sedatives.

B. Physiology and pharmacology

There are physiologic differences in infants and children that directly affect the metabolism and action of sedatives. The compartment percentages of the body vary with age. Total-body water decreases from more than 80% in preterm infants to about 60% in adults. The high total-body water creates a larger volume of distribution for water-soluble drugs in infants and younger children. Because of the larger volume of distribution, an initial **larger** dose of drug is needed to attain a similar blood level, and the excretion of a drug is delayed, requiring increased dosing intervals in neonates. Infants also have less fat and muscle compared with children and adults. Those drugs that are dependent on redistribution into fatty tissue for their termination of action have a **longer** clinical effect, which further increases the dosing interval.

There are also anatomic differences in infants and children that should be considered when preparing for procedural sedation. The central nervous system is underdeveloped in infants and is relatively predisposed to seizures and increased intracranial pressure, with subsequent potential development of intraventricular hemorrhage. The parasympathetic nervous system is particularly active in infants, whereas the sympathetic nervous system is underdeveloped. Infants have decreased glomerular filtration rate, which leads to decreased renal drug clearance. In addition, infants have decreased hepatic drug clearance because of the immature cytochrome P-450 and glucuronyl transferases. Relative to adults, infants and children have a reduced pulmonary reserve. They also have high metabolic rates and oxygen consumption. These airway differences make them more vulnerable to medications that produce hypoventilation and apnea.

C. Preparation

1. Procedural sedation is used for diagnostic studies such as neuroimaging, minor surgical procedures such as suturing, noninvasive

procedures such as fracture reduction, and invasive procedures such as drainage of abscesses. The goals of sedation are to:

a. Ensure patient safety.
b. Minimize physical discomfort and pain.
c. Minimize negative psychological responses.
d. Maximize the production of amnesia.
e. Ensure rapid recovery to the presedation level of function.

2. This is most readily accomplished in an appropriate facility and with personnel who have appropriate levels of experience.

3. Nonpharmacologic interventions may be valuable in the care of pediatric patients and should serve as adjuncts to pharmacologic agents. These nonpharmacologic interventions should be tailored to the patient's age and developmental level. They are used to relieve fear and anxiety. Examples of these interventions include pacifiers, breast-feeding, and swaddling for infants, parental holding for toddlers, and family presence and distraction with music or humor in older children.

4. An emergency care cart must be accessible and contain age- and weight-appropriate drugs and equipment to rescue a patient undergoing sedation who has an adverse event. The drugs and equipment suggested by the American Academy of Pediatrics are listed in Boxes 7-1 and 7-2.

BOX 7-1

SUGGESTED EMERGENCY DRUGS

Oxygen
Glucose (50%)
Atropine
Epinephrine (1:1,000; 1:10,000)
Phenylephrine
Dopamine
Diazepam
Isoproterenol
Calcium chloride or calcium gluconate
Sodium bicarbonate
Lidocaine (cardiac and local infiltration)
Naloxone hydrochloride
Diphenhydramine hydrochloride
Hydrocortisone
Methylprednisolone
Succinylcholine
Aminophylline
Racemic epinephrine
Albuterol by inhalation
Ammonia spirits

Note: The choice of emergency drugs would vary according to individual need.

BOX 7-2

SUGGESTED EMERGENCY EQUIPMENT

Intravenous equipment: IV catheters of varying sizes, tourniquets, assorted sized syringes, skin cleansing agent, adhesive dressing

Intravenous tubing: pediatric drip at 60 drops/mL, pediatric burette type, adult drip at 10 drops/mL, extension tubing

Intravenous fluid: Lactated Ringer's solution, normal saline

Pediatric IV boards

Intraosseous bone marrow needle

Airway management equipment: face masks, breathing bag and valve set, oral airways, nasal airways, laryngoscope handles and blades, endotracheal tubes of varying size that are uncuffed and cuffed, stylettes, surgical lubricant, suction catheters, nasogastric tubes, nebulizer with medication kits

D. Choice of agents

The ideal drug for procedural sedation would have a rapid onset, short duration, minimal adverse effects, and rapid metabolism to inactive metabolites to prevent cumulative effect.

The pharmacologic agents available for pediatric sedation include the same topical, local, and regional anesthetics and nonparenteral and parenteral agents available in adult cases. It is important that all drugs be administered in small, incremental doses with adequate time between doses to assess the full pharmacologic effect.

Since this ideal drug does not exist, a combination of drugs may be used to achieve the ideal outcome. Drug combinations utilize synergistic effects and reduce the total amount of each drug administered. This synergism is not completely predictable, and the patients must always be monitored for respiratory depression, hypoxia, and prolonged sedation. When a combination of drugs is being administered, it is prudent to begin with the lowest dosage for each and titrate to the desired clinical effect.

The sedatives typically used for pediatric sedation include chloral hydrate, benzodiazepines, barbiturates, opioids, ketamine, and propofol and are listed in Table 7-4.

1. **Etomidate:** Limited data are available regarding the use of etomidate for procedural sedation in children. Etomidate is a hypnotic with a favorable hemodynamic profile and should be considered in extreme situations.

2. **Chloral hydrate:** This is a commonly administered nonbarbiturate sedative-hypnotic that can be given orally and rectally. It is rapidly absorbed from the GI tract and is generally considered to be safe. Its duration can be prolonged, especially in neonates, because of an extended half-life and active metabolites. Adverse effects include

TABLE 7-4

AGENTS FOR PEDIATRIC SEDATION

Drug	Route of Administration	Dosage Guidelines	Adverse Events	Comments
Chloral hydrate	PO, PR	25–75 mg/kg with max. 1–2 g; max. in neonates, 50 mg/kg Give 1 hr before procedure.	Oversedation; gastrointestinal upset; respiratory depression	Available in 250- and 500-mg capsules and in 250 and 500 mg/5 mL solutions; suppositories in 325, 500, and 650 mg
Benzodiazepines			Respiratory depression; hypotension	Caution in patients who are also receiving opioids; effects can be reversed with flumazenil
Midazolam	IV, IM, PO, SL, nasal	0.05 mg/kg IV with max. 4 mg; 0.05–0.15 mg/kg IM with max. 5 mg; 0.5 mg/kg PO with max. 15 mg; 0.2 mg/kg SL or nasal with max. 5 mg	See above	Water soluble; longer onset of action when not given IV or IM
Diazepam	IV, PO	0.1–0.3 mg/kg with max. 10 mg	See above	Not water soluble
Lorazepam	IV, IM, PO	0.025–0.05 mg/kg with max. 2 mg	See above	Not water soluble; slow onset of action
Barbiturates			Respiratory depression, hypotension	
Pentobarbital	IV (slow), IM, PO, PR	1–6 mg/kg IV with max. 100 mg; 2–6 mg/kg IM, PO, PR with max. 100 mg	See above	Can have prolonged sedation; available in capsule, elixir, suppository, and injection

Thiopental	IV (slow), PR	3–6 mg/kg IV; 25–50 mg/kg PR	See above	Can have prolonged sedation
Methohexital	IV for adults, PR	0.5– 2 mg/kg IV; 20–30 mg/kg PR	See above	Available in 500-mg vial
Opioids			Respiratory depression, hypotension	Can be reversed with naloxone; no amnestic properties
Fentanyl	IV	0.5–3.0 µg/kg	See above	Note units because very potent
Morphine	IV, IM	0.05–0.15 mg/kg	See above	See above
Meperidine	IV, IM	0.5–1 mg/kg with max. 100 mg	See above	See above
Ketamine	IV, IM	0.5–2 mg/kg IV; 2–5 mg/kg IM 5–10 mg PO	Excessive salivation and airway secretions; gastrointestinal upset	Will maintain airway reflexes; bronchodilator
Propofol	IV	1.0–3.5 mg/kg	Respiratory depression, hypotension	Titrate to desired effect; watch for adverse effects

IM, intramuscular; IV, intravenous; PO, oral; PR, rectal; SL, sublingual.

PEDIATRIC CONSIDERATIONS 7

respiratory depression, hypotension, prolonged sedation, disorientation, and GI upset.

3. **Benzodiazepines:** These are a class of sedative-hypnotics that act at the γ-aminobutyric acid A (GABA-A) receptor complex. Midazolam is the most commonly prescribed drug in this class and can be administered orally, intranasally, rectally, intramuscularly, and intravenously. It has potent amnestic and anxiolytic properties and is short-acting. There are no analgesic properties. Adverse effects include respiratory depression, hypotension, and vasodilation. The hypotensive effect is worsened in patients with hypovolemia. Using the antagonist flumazenil can reverse respiratory depression.

4. **Barbiturates:** These are a class of sedative hypnotics that depress the reticular activating system by inhibiting the dissociation of GABA from the GABA-A receptor complex. Barbiturates are distributed in the body on the basis of their lipid solubility, protein binding, and extent to which they are ionized. They have no analgesic properties. They are metabolized in the liver, and the metabolites are water soluble and excreted through the kidneys. The barbiturates used for sedation are the ultra-short- and short-acting agents that can be administered orally, rectally, intramuscularly, and intravenously. Adverse effects include respiratory depression, hypotension, and delirium.

5. **Opioids:** These are often used in conjunction with a sedative to achieve analgesia for painful procedures. Care must be exercised in this situation because of the synergistic respiratory depression with sedatives. Other adverse effects include nausea, vomiting, and hypotension. Naloxone can be used to reverse the respiratory depression caused by opioids.

6. **Ketamine:** This agent is a dissociative agent that produces analgesia as well as amnesia and sedation. It has a rapid onset of action when administered in the preferred intramuscular or intravenous form. It can be given orally and rectally, but has less predictable effectiveness and requires substantially higher doses. Protective airway reflexes are **usually** preserved with ketamine, and spontaneous respirations are almost always maintained. It does produce excessive salivation and airway secretion and has been associated with laryngospasm. Although ketamine has been associated with emergence dysphonia and hallucinations in adults, this phenomenon does not appear to be prominent in children.

7. **Propofol:** This is a very short-acting sedative-hypnotic nonbarbiturate with anxiolytic and antiemetic properties. It has no analgesic properties. It has a rapid onset of action and is titratable. Propofol can cause severe pain at the injection site, which can be minimized by injecting into a large vein or by mixing with lidocaine. Other adverse effects include hypotension, respiratory depression, and dysphoric reactions.

III. EXTREMELY HANDY PEDIATRIC INFORMATION

A. Fasting guidelines
1. Clear liquids have been shown not to increase the risk for aspiration (no difference in gastric residual volume or pH) when given in unlimited quantity up to 2 hours before surgery as compared with 6 to 8 hours.
2. In contrast, milk and formula have similar risk as solids; hence, NPO status is the same.
3. Breast milk is unclear and is treated at a risk intermediate between clear liquids and formula.
4. Current guidelines are shown in Table 7-5.

B. Routine preprocedure labs
1. Infants < 6 months of age: depends on patient's physiologic status; may need heelstick hematocrit—discuss with faculty
2. Children > 6 months of age: no routine labs for otherwise healthy children
3. Always adjust this guideline depending on illness severity and procedure planned.

C. Premedication
1. Purpose: to help with a traumatic separation from parents
2. Variety available: including midazolam (intranasal, rectal, PO) methohexital/pentobarbital (rectal), ketamine (IM)
3. Consider premedicating all patients older than 12 months unless there is contraindication to sedation. A useful premedication is oral midazolam, 0.5 mg/kg (up to 20 mg), mixed with Tylenol.

D. Latex allergy
1. At-risk groups: patients with spina bifida, congenital urologic abnormalities (bladder extrophy), history of atopy (ABC) allergies (avocado, banana, chestnut), health care worker
2. Latex anaphylaxis:
a. Onset within 30 minutes after exposure to antigen (range, 5 to 290 minutes)
b. Presents as rash, hypotension, bronchospasm

E. Treatment of anaphylaxis
1. Remove antigen if detected
2. 100% oxygen

TABLE 7-5

FASTING GUIDELINES

Age	Clear Liquids*	Breast Milk	Milk, Formula, Solids
0–6 mo	2 hr	4 hr	8 hr
>6 mo	2 hr	4 hr	8 hr

*May use 3 hours to give leeway for change of schedules.

3. Intravenous fluids
4. Adjust or discontinue anesthetics
5. Discontinue antibiotic infusion or blood product transfusion if in progress
6. Antihistamine
a. Diphenhydramine: 1 mg/kg IV (max. 100 mg)
b. Cimetidine: 5 to 7.5 mg/kg IV (max. 300 mg)
7. Steroids
a. Dexamethasone: 0.3 mg/kg IV (max. 10 mg)
b. Hydrocortisone: 2 mg/kg IV (max. 100 mg)
c. Methylprednisolone: 5 mg/kg IV (max. 125 mg)
8. Epinephrine
a. For bronchospasm: infusion at 0.5 to 1 μg/kg per minute
b. For hypotension: bolus, begin at 1 to 2 μg/kg
c. For cardiac arrest: bolus, begin at 10 μg/kg

F. Considerations of prematurity

1. Retinopathy of prematurity

Note: *Etiology is multifactorial, and hyperoxia is one factor.*

a. Safe Pao_2 thought to be 50 to 70 mm Hg
b. Corresponding Spo_2 90 to 95
c. At-risk patients: up to 44 weeks postconceptional age
d. Exacerbated by hypercarbia, hypocarbia
2. Postprocedure apnea guidelines
a. Delay procedure if possible until postconceptional age > 50 weeks.
b. Regional anesthesia if possible—no sedative drugs.
c. If general anesthesia, then consider caffeine, 10 mg/kg IV after
   induction, if not taking theophylline.
d. Former preterm infants, postconceptional age < 50 weeks, admit for
   minimum of 23 apnea-free hours, regardless of anesthesia type.
e. Former preterm infants, postconceptional age > 50 weeks, monitor for
   2 apnea-free hours before discharging from postanesthetic care unit.
f. Patients with significant coexisting disease (history of apnea, chronic
   lung disease, anemia, neurologic deficit) require an individualized plan.
g. Full term infants, postconceptional age < 44 weeks, admit for 12 hours
   minimum, regardless of anesthesia type.
3. Definitions:
a. Periodic breathing = 5 to 10 seconds of no airflow (no bradycardia or
   hypoxemia; *can be normal*)
b. Apnea ≥ 20 seconds of no airflow
   (1) < 20 seconds of no airflow with bradycardia or hypoxemia
   (2) Postconceptional age < 37 weeks at birth and weighs < 2500 g.

G. Temperature

See Table 7-6.

TABLE 7-6

TEMPERATURE

	Premature	Term	Adult
Neutral temperature*	34° C	32° C	28° C
Critical temperature[†]	28° C	23° C	1° C

*Ambient room temperature resulting in minimal O_2 consumption.
[†]Ambient temperature below which an unclothed, unanesthetized patient cannot maintain a normal core temperature.

1. Use the Warm Touch heating blanket for all patients < 1 year old or < 10 kg. Be careful that the heating hose does not touch the lower extremities.
2. Must measure core temperature when using heating blanket (not axillary).
3. Set room thermostat in advance to at least:
a. 80° F for neonates
b. 78° F for infants
c. 76° F for children 6 to 24 months old
4. Neonates and infants tend to lose body heat rapidly:
a. Large body surface area relative to body weight
b. Little subcutaneous fat
c. Decreased ability to produce heat

H. Cardiovascular physiology
See Table 7-7.

I. Fluids and chemistry
See Table 7-8.

J. Blood product composition
See Table 7-9.

K. Normal screening tests
See Table 7-10.

TABLE 7-7

CARDIOVASCULAR PHYSIOLOGY

Age	Weight (kg)	Heart Rate (beats/min)	Normal Blood Pressure (mm Hg)	Blood Volume (mL/kg)
Premature	1.0	120–180	40/20	90–100
Term	3.0	95–145	60/35	80–90
1 mo	4.0*	100–140	75/40	80
6 mo	7.0[†]	110–180	90/40	75–80
1 yr	10	100–160	95/50	75
5 yr	20	65–135	100/60	70–75
Adult	70	50–95	120/70	70

TABLE 7-8

FLUIDS AND CHEMISTRY

Age	Premature	Term	1 yr	2 yr	Adult
Extracellular fluid (% body weight)	50	35–40	30	<30	20
Intracellular fluid (% body weight)	30	35	35	>35	45
Na^+	133–146	136–148	135–145	135–145	135–145
K^+	4.6–6.7	4.3–7.6	3.5–5.5	3.5–5.5	3.5–5.5
Cl^-	100–117	90–114	94–105	94–105	94–105
HCO_3^-	20	22	20–25	20–25	22–26
Total calcium	6–10	7–12	8–11	8.5–10.5	8.5–10.5
Glucose	40–65	40–110	60–105	60–105	60–105
Total protein	3.9–4.7	4.6–7.7		5.5–7.8	5.5–7.8
Blood urea nitrogen	9	13	5.25	5.25	5.25
Creatinine	<0.5	<0.5	0.5–0.6	0.5–0.9	0.5–1.2
Glomerular filtration rate $(mL/min/1.73\ m^2)$	13–58	15–60	60–120	120	120
Max. mOsm/L	400–600	400–600	1400	1400	1400

L. Intubation

See Table 7-11.

1. Endotracheal tube (ETT) tube formulas (none are perfect)
a. ETT size in internal diameter (ID) (mm) = (age ÷ 4) + 4
b. Depth—oral (cm) at lips = (age ÷ 2) + 13 = 3 × ETT size
c. 50 percentile wt (kg) = 9 + (2 × age)
2. Laryngeal mask airway (Table 7-12)

TABLE 7-9

BLOOD PRODUCT COMPOSITION

	Normal	Citrated Whole Blood	Citrated Packed Red Blood Cells	Fresh Frozen Plasma
pH	74	≅6.8	≅6.8	≅6.8
P_{CO_2}	40	≅190	≅190	≅190
Base deficit mEq/L	0	≅12	≅12	≅12
K^+ mEq/L	3.5–5.0	>18	>18	4–8
Citrate	—	++	+	+++
Factors V and VIII	Normal	<20%	—	80–100%
Fibrinogen	Normal	—	—	—
Platelets	160–400K	—	—	—
2,3-DPG	Normal	3%	3%	—
Hct	35–45	35–45	70–80	—
Temperature (°C)	37	1–6	1–6	Cold

TABLE 7-10

NORMAL SCREENING TESTS

Test	Preterm Newborn (<1500 g)	Preterm Newborn (1500–2000 g)	Full-Term Newborn	Adult
Platelet count (10^3, mm^3)	250 (>150)	250 (>150)	250 (>150)	300 (>150)
PTT (sec)	108 (<150)	80 (<120)	65 (<84)	44 (<50)
PT (sec)	17 (<20)	16 (<19)	13.5 (<16)	12 (<14)
INR*	<2.3	<2.0	<1.4	<1.1
Thrombin time (sec)	15 (<20)	15 (<20)	14 (<18)	10 (<12)

*International normalized ratio.

3. Notes on intubation and ETT selection
a. Leak pressure
    (1) Important to check because the narrowest portion is at the cricoid ring instead of the vocal cords (up to 7 to 9 years of age)
    (2) Document, with goal of 20 to 30 cm H_2O
b. Reintubation within 1 month—always compare leak with previous value to eliminate the beginning of edema and stenosis.
c. Always avoid endobronchial intubation.
d. Resistance:
    (1) Resistance $= 8lv/r^4$, where $l =$ length, $v =$ viscosity, $r =$ radius; related to $1/radius^4$ and length (Poiseuille's law)
    (2) Changing from 3.5 to 3.0 mm ID ETT increases resistance by nearly 50%.
    (3) Changing from 7.5 to 7.0 mm ID ETT increases resistance by 24%.
    (4) Turbulent flow exists at sites of luminal change (secretions and kinks) and adds to the resistance to laminar flow.
e. In tubes of appropriate length:
    (1) 3.5 ETT offers less resistance than the normal neonatal airway.
    (2) 2.5 ETT offers more resistance than the natural airway.
f. Cuffed tubes:
    (1) Cuffed ETTs are rarely necessary in children younger than 8 to 10 years. The addition of a cuff increases the outer diameter of an ETT; therefore, when a cuff is needed, the estimated tube size should be reduced by 0.5 mm ID.
    (2) Recent studies show no increased complication rates with cuffed ETTs. Advantages of a cuffed ETT include avoidance of repeated laryngoscopy and thus less airway trauma, use of low fresh gas flow, and reduction of the concentration of anesthetics detected in the operating room.

M. Pediatric airway differences
1. Head: occiput is large, may give natural sniffing position
2. Tongue: larger in relation to pharynx

TABLE 7-11

INTUBATION BLADES

	Miller 0		Miller 1		Mac 2	WH 1.5*	Mac 3 / Miller 2	
Age	Premature	Term	3 mo	1 yr	3 yr	5 yr	10 yr	Adult
Weight (kg)	1	2	3	5	11	15	19	35	70
ETT size ID (mm)	2.5	2.5–	3.0–	3.5	4.0	4.5	5.0	5.5	8.0–
Depth								
oral (cm)	7	8	9	10.5	12	13.5	15	18	19–23
nasal (cm)	9	9	9–10	12	14	17	19	22–24	25–31

*WH 1.5 = Wis-Hipple 1.5 for ages 2–4 years.

ETT, endotracheal tube; ID, internal diameter.

TABLE 7-12

LARYNGEAL MASK AIRWAY

Mask Size	Patient Weight (kg)	Cuff Volume (mL)	FOB size (OD, mm)	Largest ETT (ID, mm)
1	<5	<4	2.7	3.5
1.5	5–10	<7	3.0	4.0
2	10–20	<10	3.5	4.5
2.5	20–30	<14	4.0	5.0
3	30–50	<20	5.0	6.0 cuffed
4	50–70	<30	5.0	6.0 cuffed
5	<70	<40	7.3	7.0 cuffed

ETT, endotracheal tube; FOB, fiberoptic bronchoscope; OD, outside diameter.

3. Epiglottis: narrow, omega-shaped, protruding
4. Hyoid bone: not calcified
5. Larynx: higher C3–4 (adult = C5–6) angulated, anterior
6. Thyroid cartilage: not calcified
7. Cricoid cartilage: conical, narrowest point of airway below 10 years
8. Trachea: deviated down and posterior
9. Obligate nasal breathers

N. Extubation
1. Postextubation stridor
a. Usually within 1 hour of extubation
b. Associated with prolonged intubation, multiple head movements, tight-fitting tube, traumatic intubation, history of stridor or croup, presence of upper respiratory infection
c. Ages 1 to 4 years (not exclusively)
d. Treatment
   (1) Racemic epinephrine: 0.25 to 0.5 mL; dilute to 3 mL with normal saline and humidified oxygen on air
   (2) Decadron: 1 to 4 mg IV
2. Laryngospasm
a. Usually shortly after extubation (can also occur during induction, intraoperative with a laryngeal mask airway (LMA) or accidental extubation)
b. Associated with stage II and unnoticed partial upper airway obstruction
c. Treatment
   (1) 100% O_2 via face mask
   (2) Gentle positive pressure
   (3) Succinylcholine: 0.25 to 1 mg/kg IV; 4 to 6 mg/kg IV
   (4) Lidocaine: 1 to 1.5 mg/kg IV may help.

O. Regional anesthesia
1. Spinal anesthesia for neonates, infants who were premature
a. Neonatal spinal needle, 22 g, short bevel

b. L4–5 interspace, no higher

c. Inject slowly.

d. Use tuberculin syringe.

e. Add volume for dead space of needle.

f. Hold needle in for 5 seconds after injection complete.

g. 0.5% tetracaine in D5W (5% dextrose) = equal volumes of 1% tetracaine in water + D10W (10% dextrose solution)

h. Premature: 0.8 to 1.0 mg/kg

i. Minimum dose: 1 mg

j. Rapid T2 to T4 block; lasts 45 to 60 minutes. Block starts to wear off by 45 minutes. Cannot count on longer duration; be sure that surgeon is aware of the time limit, and this includes prep time.

2. Caudal analgesia

a. Landmarks for caudal analgesia are easily palpable in infants and prepubertal children.

b. Level with volume of anesthetic

    (1) Armitage formula: bupivacaine: 0.125% to 0.25% ± epinephrine

        (a) Lumbar: 0.5 mL/kg

        (b) Low thoracic: 1.0 mL/kg

        (c) Midthoracic: 1.25 mL/kg

    (2) Spear formula:

        (a) Midthoracic: 1.6 mL/kg

        (b) Percentage concentration: tradeoff between motor and sensory block

3. Epidural analgesia for local anesthetic/opioid mixtures (Table 7-13)

4. Lumbar and caudal epidural opioids

a. Morphine bolus: 30 to 40 µg/kg q 8 to 12 hours

b. Fentanyl bolus: 50 to 100 µg (1 to 2 µg/kg)

5. Intrathecal morphine: 10 to 20 µg/kg intrathecal

6. Epidural and intrathecal narcotics—side effects and treatments

a. Respiratory depression

    (1) Fio_2 ± assisted ventilation

    (2) Naloxone: 5 µg/kg IV push

    (3) Reduce or discontinue infusion

b. Pruritus

    (1) Naloxone: 5 µg/kg IV push

    (2) Diphenhydramine: 0.125 to 0.25 mg/kg IV every 6 hours up to 25 mg

TABLE 7-13

EPIDURAL ANALGESIA

Age	Bolus (mL/kg/segment)	Infusion (Starting Rate) (mL/kg/hr)
<1 yr	0.04–0.05	0.1–0.2*
1–7 yr	0.03–0.04	0.1–0.4†
>7 yr	0.02–0.03	0.1–0.4†

*Bupivacaine 0.1% + 3 µg/mL fentanyl.
†Bupivacaine 0.1% + 10 µg/mL fentanyl.

(3) Propofol: 0.1 mg/kg × one bolus, may repeat once at 15 minutes
(4) Reduce dose of narcotic bolus or decrease infusion rate
c. Nausea ± vomiting
(1) Metoclopramide: 0.15 mg/kg every 8 hours
(2) Dolasetron: 0.35 mg/kg IV every 8 hours up to 12 mg
(3) Propofol (as above)
(4) Naloxone: 5 µg/kg IV push
(5) NPO
d. Urinary retention
(1) Straight catheter
(2) Naloxone: 5 µg/kg IV push

P. Pharmacology
1. Antibiotics—intravenous (Table 7-14)
a. Gentamicin for neonates < 7 days old:
(1) < 28 weeks postconceptional age: 2.5 mg/kg per day every
24 hours
(2) 28 to 34 weeks postconceptional age: 2.5 mg/kg per day every
18 hours
(3) Term: 2.5 mg/kg per day every 12 hours
b. Gentamicin for neonates > 7 days old:
(1) < 23 weeks postconceptional age: 2.5 mg/kg per day every 18 hours
(2) 28 to 34 weeks: 2.5 mg/kg per day every 12 hours
(3) Term: 2.5 mg/kg per day every 8 hours
2. Anticonvulsants (status epilepticus dosing)
a. Diazepam
(1) 1 month to 5 years old: 0.2 to 0.5 mg/kg IV every 10 to
30 minutes; max. 5 mg
(2) > 5 years old: 1.0 mg IV every 15 to 30 minutes; max. 10 mg
b. Phenobarbital
(1) 10 to 20 mg/kg/dose IV × 1, then 5 to 10 mg/kg/dose every
20 minutes as needed
(2) Max. total dose: 40 mg/kg
c. Phenytoin
(1) 15 to 20 mg/kg IV load (slow); max. 1 g/24 hours
(2) Therapeutic levels: 10 to 20 µg/mL

TABLE 7-14

INTRAVENOUS ANTIBIOTICS

Single Intraoperative Doses		Max (Adult)	Total Daily Dose
Ampicillin	50–100 mg/kg	2 g	200–400 mg/kg/day
Cefazolin	25–40 mg/kg	1 g	200 mg/kg/day
Cefotetan	20–30 mg/kg	1 g	40–60 mg/kg/day
Cefuroxime	25–50 mg/kg	0.750–1.5 g	50–100 mg/kg/day
Clindamycin	5–10 mg/kg	300 mg	15–40 mg/kg/day
Gentamicin	2 mg/kg	100 mg	5–7 mg/kg/day

3. Antidysrhythmics
a. Bretylium
   (1) IV: 5 mg/kg over 1 minute, then 5 to 10 mg/kg every 15 to
      30 minutes
   (2) Max. 30 mg/kg
b. Esmolol
   (1) IV: 0.2 to 0.5 mg/kg IV push
   (2) Load: 0.5 mg/kg
   (3) Infusion: 50 to 200 μg/kg per minute
c. Labetalol
   (1) IV: 0.125 to 0.25 mg/kg
d. Lidocaine
   (1) IV load: 1.0 mg/kg, repeat to max. 3 to 5 mg/kg
   (2) Infusion: 30 to 50 μg/kg per minute
e. Phenytoin
   (1) IV: 2 to 4 mg/kg over 5 minutes, up to 15 mg/kg
f. Procainamide
   (1) IV load: 2 to 5 mg/kg over 30 minutes
   (2) Infusion: 20 to 80 μg/kg per minute; max. 50 to 60 mg/kg
      per day
g. Adenosine IV
4. Antiemetics
a. Droperidol IV: 10 to 70 μg/kg (**Beware:** Recent FDA Black Box warning)
b. Metoclopramide IV: 0.15 mg/kg, max. 10 mg
c. Ondansetron IV: 0.15 mg/kg, max. 4 mg
d. Dolasetron IV: 0.35 mg/kg, max. 12.5 mg
5. Bronchodilators
a. Albuterol: inhaled, usually 2.5 mg in 2.5 mL normal saline, given to all
   patients (for premature infants, may use 1.25 mg).
b. Aminophylline
   (1) IV: 6 mg/kg slow IV push load (over 30 minutes)
   (2) IV: 0.2 to 1.0 mg/kg per hour (therapeutic level 10 to 20 mg/L)
c. Dexamethasone: IV, 0.25 to 1.0 mg/kg load
d. Epinephrine: SC, 0.01 mL/kg (1:1000); max. 0.5 mL
e. Hydrocortisone
   (1) IV: 4 to 8 mg/kg load
   (2) IV: 8 mg/kg per 24 hours, infuse or divided every 6 hours
f. Metaproterenol: inhaled, 0.2 to 0.3 mL in 2.5 mL saline via
   nebulizer
g. Methylprednisolone
   (1) IV: 1 to 2 mg/kg load
   (2) 1.6 mg/kg per 24 hours, divided every 6 hours
6. Diuretics
a. Furosemide: 1 mg/kg IV
b. Mannitol: 0.25 to 1 g/kg IV
7. Epinephrine dilutions

a. 1:10,000 = 100 µg/mL
b. 1:100,000 = 10 µg/mL
c. 1:200,000 = 5 µg/mL
d. 1:400,000 = 2.5 µg/mL
8. H_2 blockers, antacids
   a. Cimetidine IV/PO: 20 to 40 mg/kg per day, divided every 6 hours, max. 300 mg/dose
   b. Famotidine IV/PO: 1 to 2 mg/kg per day, divided every 12 hours, max. 40 mg/dose
   c. Ranitidine
      (1) IV: 1 to 2 mg/kg per day divided every 6 hours, max. 50 mg/dose
      (2) PO: 2 to 4 mg/kg per day divided every 12 hours, max. 150 mg/dose
   d. Sodium citrate PO: 0.4 mL/kg, max. 30 mL
9. Induction-sedative agents
   a. Chloral hydrate PO/PR: 50 to 70 mg/kg (hypnotic dose), max. 1 g/dose
   b. Diazepam IV: 0.05 to 0.3 mg/kg
   c. Etomidate IV: 0.2 to 0.3 mg/kg
   d. Ketamine
      (1) IV: 1 to 2 mg/kg
      (2) IM/PO: 5 to 10 mg/kg
   e. Methohexital
      (1) IV: 0.5 to 2 mg/kg
      (2) Rectal: 30 mg/kg
   f. Midazolam
      (1) IV: 0.02 to 0.05 mg/kg
      (2) PO: 0.5 to 1.0 mg/kg
   g. Propofol
      (1) IV: 2.5 to 3.5 mg/kg
      (2) Infusion: 50 to 200 µg/kg per minute
   h. Thiopental
      (1) IV: 3 to 6 mg/kg
      (2) Rectal: 20 to 30 mg/kg
10. Benzodiazepine antagonist: flumazenil IV: 8 to 15 µg/kg, titrated to effect
11. Inotropes and vasopressors
    a. Digoxin: total digitalizing dose (TDD): give ½ TDD slow IV push, then ¼ TDD IV every 6 hours × 2.
       (1) Premature: 20 µg//kg
       (2) Neonate: 30 µg/kg
       (3) < 2 years: 30 to 50 µg/kg
       (4) 2 to 10 years: 15 to 30 µg/kg
       (5) > 10 years: 10 to 15 µg/kg
       (6) Therapeutic levels: 0.8 to 2.0 µg/L
    b. Dobutamine IV: 1 to 10 µg/kg per minute, max. 40 µg/kg per minute
    c. Dopamine IV: 1 to 20 µg/kg per minute

d. Epinephrine IV: 0.1 to 1.0 µg/kg per minute
e. Milrinone
  (1) IV load: 50 µg/kg over 10 minutes
  (2) Infusion: 0.375 to 0.750 µg/kg per minute
f. Norepinephrine IV: 0.1 to 1.0 µg/kg per minute
g. Phenylephrine IV: 0.1 to 1.0 µg/kg per minute
12. IV push doses
a. Ephedrine: 0.1 mg/kg
b. Epinephrine: 1 to 10 µg/kg
c. Phenylephrine: 1 to 2 µg/kg

Q. Pediatric resuscitation doses

See Table 7-15.
1. Muscle relaxants—intubating doses
a. *cis*-Atracurium IV: 0.1 mg/kg
b. Mivacurium IV: 0.2 mg/kg
c. Pancuronium IV: 0.1 mg/kg
d. Rapacuronium—removed from the market due to bronchospasm risks.
e. Rocuronium IV: 0.6 to 1.2 mg/kg
f. Succinylcholine
  (1) IV: 1 to 2 mg/kg
  (2) IM: 4 to 5 mg/kg
g. Vecuronium IV: 0.1 mg/kg
2. Reversal agents and adjuncts
a. Edrophonium (IV: 0.5 to 1 mg/kg) and atropine (IV: 15 to 20 µg/kg)
b. Neostigmine (IV: 50 to 70 µg/kg) and glycopyrrolate (15 µg/kg) (EQUAL VOLUMES OF EACH)
3. Narcotics
a. Alfentanil
  (1) IV load: 30 to 50 µg/kg
  (2) Infusion: 0.5 to 1.5 µg/kg per minute

TABLE 7-15

PEDIATRIC RESUSCITATION DOSES

Drug	Route	Dose
Atropine	IV	20 µg/kg
Epinephrine	IV	10 µg/kg
Calcium chloride	IV	20 mg/kg
Lidocaine	IV	1 mg/kg (every 5–10 min to 4 mg/kg)
Dextrose	IV	0.5 g/kg
Naloxone	IV	10 µg/kg
Na bicarbonate	IV	1–2 mEq/kg (4.2%)
Bretylium	IV	5 mg/kg (5–10 mg/kg every 10 min, <17 mg/kg)
Defibrillation		2 J/kg, then 4 J/kg

b. Fentanyl IV: 1 to 5 µg/kg
c. Meperidine IV: 1 to 2 mg/kg
d. Morphine IV: 0.1 to 0.2 mg/kg
e. Sufentanil IV:0.1–1 ug/kg
   (1) IV load: 2 to 10 µg/kg
   (2) Infusion: 0.1 to 0.5 µg/kg per minute
f. Remifentanil
   (1) IV load: 0.5 to 2.0 µg/kg
   (2) Infusion: 0.05 to 2.0 µg/kg per minute
4. Narcotic antagonist: naloxone IV: 5 to 10 µg/kg, repeat every 3 to 5 minutes
5. Parasympathetic antagonists
a. Atropine IV/IM: 10 to 20 µg/kg
b. Glycopyrrolate IV: 5 to 10 µg/kg
c. Scopolamine IV: 5 to 10 µg/kg
6. Steroids
a. Dexamethasone IV: 0.3 to 1.0 mg/kg (load)
b. Hydrocortisone IV: 2 mg/kg every 6 hours
7. Vasodilators
a. Labetalol IV: 0.125 to 0.25 mg/kg
b. Nitroglycerin IV: 0.5 to 10 µg/kg per minute
c. Phentolamine
   (1) IV: 50 to 100 µg/kg
   (2) Infusion: 10 to 20 µg/kg per minute
d. Prostaglandin E_1 IV: 0.1 µg/kg per minute
e. Sodium nitroprusside IV: 0.5 to 10 µg/kg per minute
8. Miscellaneous
a. Dantrolene IV: 2.5 mg/kg to 10 mg/kg max.
b. Dextrose IV: 0.25 to 0.5 g/kg IV (= 2 mL/kg of 25% dextrose)
c. Diphenhydramine IV: 0.125 to 0.25 mg/kg every 6 hours
d. Insulin IV: 0.02 to 0.1 U/kg per hour
e. Calcium gluconate IV: 30 mg/kg

R. Subacute bacterial endocarditis (SBE) prophylactic regimens
1. Goals of prophylactic regimens: Prophylaxis is most effective when given in doses that are sufficient to ensure adequate antibiotic concentrations in the serum during and after the procedure. To reduce the likelihood of microbial resistance, it is important that prophylactic antibiotics be used only during the periprocedure period. They should be initiated shortly before a procedure and should not be continued for an extended period (no more than 6 to 8 hours) (Table 7-16).
2. Regimens for genitourinary and nonesophageal GI procedures: Antibiotic prophylaxis to prevent endocarditis should be directed primarily against enterococci (Table 7-17).

TABLE 7-16

PROPHYLACTIC REGIMENS FOR DENTAL, ORAL, RESPIRATORY TRACT, OR ESOPHAGEAL PROCEDURES

Situation	Agent	Regimen*
Standard general prophylaxis	Amoxicillin	50 mg/kg PO, max. 2.0 g, 1 hr before procedure
Unable to take oral medications	Ampicillin	50 mg/kg IM/IV, max. 2.0 g, 30 min before procedure
Allergic to penicillin	Clindamycin, *or*	20 mg/kg PO, up to 600 mg, 1hr before procedure
	Cephalexin,† *or*	50 mg/kg PO, max. 2.0 g, 1 hr before procedure
	Azithromycin	15 mg/kg PO, up to 500 mg, 1 hr before procedure
Allergic to penicillin and unable to take oral	Clindamycin, *or*	20 mg/kg IV, up to 600 mg, 30 min before procedure
medications	Cefazolin†	25 mg/kg IM/IV, up to 1.0 g, 30 min before procedure

*No follow-up doses recommended.

†Cephalosporins should not be used in patients who have immediate-type hypersensitivity reaction to penicillins.

TABLE 7-17

PROPHYLACTIC REGIMENS FOR GENITOURINARY AND GASTROINTESTINAL (EXCLUDING ESOPHAGEAL) PROCEDURES

Situation	Agents	Regimen*
High-risk patients	Ampicillin plus gentamicin	Ampicillin 50 mg/kg IM/IV (max. 2.0 g) plus gentamycin 1.5 mg/kg (max. 120 mg) within 30 min of starting the procedure; 6 hr later, ampicillin 25 mg/kg IM/IV or amoxicillin 25 mg/kg PO
High-risk patients allergic to ampicillin or amoxicillin	Vancomycin plus gentamicin	Vancomycin 20 mg/kg IV (max. 1 g) over 1–2 hr plus gentamycin 1.5 mg/kg (max. 120 mg) IV/IM
Moderate-risk patients	Amoxicillin or ampicillin	Amoxicillin 50 mg/kg PO (max. 2.0 g), 1 hr before procedure, or ampicillin 50 mg/kg IM/IV (max. 2.0 g) within 30 min of starting procedure
Moderate-risk patients allergic to ampicillin or amoxicillin	Vancomycin	Vancomycin 20 mg/kg IV (max. 1.0 g) over 1–2 hr complete infusion within 30 min of starting procedure

*No second dose of vancomycin or gentamicin is recommended.

BIBLIOGRAPHY

Bauman BH, McManus JG. Pediatric pain management in the emergency department. *Emerg Med Clin North Am* 2005; 23:393–414.

Committee on Drugs. Guidelines for monitoring and management of pediatric patients during and after sedation for diagnostic and therapeutic procedures. *Pediatrics* 1992; 89(6):1110–1115.

Greco C, Berde C. Pain management for the hospitalized pediatric patient. *Pediatr Clin North Am* 2005; 52:995–1027.

Krauss B, Brustowicz R (eds). *Pediatric Procedural Sedation and Analgesia*. Baltimore: Lippincott Williams & Wilkins, 1999.

Malamed S. *Sedation: A Guide to Patient Management*. St. Louis: Mosby, 2003.

Resident's Handbook of Pediatric Anesthesia. Jackson, MS, Department of Anesthesiology, University of Mississippi Medical Center.

Shankar V, Deshpande J. Procedural sedation in the pediatric patient. *Anesthesiol Clin North Am* 2005; 23(4):635–654.

Verghese ST, Hannallah RS. Postoperative pain management in children. *Anesthesiol Clin North Am* 2005; 23:163–184.

Writing Committee for the EMSC Grant Panel. Clinical policy: Evidence-based approach to pharmacologic agents used in pediatric sedation and analgesia in the emergency department. *Ann Emerg Med* 2004; 44(4):342–377.

Patient-Controlled Analgesia (PCA)

W. James Phillips

I. OVERVIEW

A. Patient-controlled analgesia (PCA) is a pain relief technique that allows selected patients to self-administer intravenous analgesics on an as-needed (PRN) basis. Parameters of dose, time interval, and cumulative dose limits are set by the practitioner.

B. Keys to success are:
1. Patient selection and education
2. Proper opiate and dose selection
3. Getting the patient to an appropriate level of analgesia by bolus therapy before starting the PCA
4. Regular reevaluation to ensure adequacy of analgesia and for surveillance of side effects
5. Realizing that "one size does not fit all" and doses and intervals must be individualized
6. The selected agent is delivered through a programmable pump with which the following parameters are programmed:
a. Patient demand dose
b. Dosing interval or lockout interval
c. Time-based cumulative dose limit (usually a 4-hour limit is used).
d. Optional basal infusion rate as background

II. TYPICAL AGENT CONCENTRATIONS
See Table 8-1.

III. TYPICAL DOSE RANGES
See Table 8-2.

IV. PCA DEMAND DOSE
A. Tables 8-1 and 8-2 provide guidelines for PCA demand doses.

B. Decrease doses for age > 70 years, hepatic dysfunction, elevated creatinine, neurologic impairment, and morbid obesity.

C. More than 3 to 4 demands per hour means inadequate analgesia.

D. Titrate dose upward in 25% increments.

E. Beware of co-administration of other sedatives.

"""

TABLE 8-1

TYPICAL AGENTS

Drug	Concentration	Bolus Dose	Demand Dose	Infusion	Lockout	4-Hour Limit
Morphine	1 mg/mL	0.05–0.15 mg/kg	0.01–0.03 mg/kg	0.01–0.03 mg/hr	10 min	±15 mg
Hydromorphone*	0.2 mg/mL	0.01–0.02 mg/kg	2–6 µg/kg	2–6 µg/kg/hr	10 min	1–2.5 mg
Meperidine	10 mg/mL	0.2–0.75 mg/kg	0.1–0.2 mg/kg	Not recommended	10–15 min	100 mg
Fentanyl[†]	20 µg/mL	1–3 µg/kg	0.1–0.5 µg/kg	0.5–1 µg/kg/hr	10 min	800 µg
Methadone	Not generally used					

*Drug of second choice in renal failure.
†Drug of choice in renal failure.

PATIENT-CONTROLLED ANALGESIA (PCA) 8

TABLE 8-2

TYPICAL DOSES

Drug	Concentration	Bolus Dose	Demand Dose	Infusion	Lockout	4-Hour Limit
Morphine	1 mg/mL	4–15 mg	0.5–3 mg	1–3 mg/hr	10 min	15 mg
Hydromorphone	0.2 mg/mL	0.5–2 mg	0.1–0.4 mg	0.1–2 mg/hr	10 min	2.5 mg
Meperidine	10 mg/mL	10–50 mg	10–20 mg	Not recommended	15 min	100 mg
Fentanyl	20 µg/mL	50–150 µg	20–40 µg	30–70 µg/hr	10 min	800 µg

F. Lockout intervals

1. This reflects the minimum time between drug delivery, regardless of the number of times the button is pressed.
2. Decreasing the lockout interval rarely helps improve analgesia.
3. Adequate time must be given to allow effects of administered drug to be felt.

G. Cumulative dose limit

1. Mentally calculate a reasonable 24-hour limit.
2. Predict the effects of any active metabolites such as normeperidine or morphine-6-glucuronide.
3. The dose limit is an added protective factor that allows higher doses in shorter dosing intervals while protecting the patient from overdose.

H. Basal infusions are:

1. Rarely useful
2. More beneficial in children than adults
3. Calculated based on giving one third of the expected hourly usage by infusion and two thirds by patient demand.
4. Many consider meperidine contraindicated for use by infusion. If used, 24-hour dose limits should be below 5 to 6 mg/kg or ± 400 to 500 mg per 24 hours.
5. Patients receiving infusions may develop tolerance more rapidly.

I. Transitioning from PCA to PO

1. Calculate the 24-hour total mg PCA use.
2. Convert this to oral equivalents.
3. Typically oral dose = 3 × IV dose for morphine, 2 × IV dose for hydromorphone
4. Give first PO doses while PCA remains in place for 8 to 12 hours to ensure good transitional analgesia.
5. If converting to long-acting opiates supplemented by breakthrough agents, allow PCA to remain in effect 24 hours after starting a patch or twice-daily longer-acting opiate.

V. MANAGING OPIATE SIDE EFFECTS

A. When writing PCA orders include:

1. PRN nausea medications
2. Scheduled constipation prophylaxis
3. Rescue medications for respiratory depression

B. PRN antiemetics

1. Promethazine (Phenergan)
a. 12.5 to 25 mg IV every 6 hours
b. 25 mg PO every 6 hours

c. Liquid 25 mg/5 mL, suppository 12.5, 25 mg
2. Prochlorperazine (Compazine)
a. 5 to 10 IV every 6 hours
b. 10 mg PO every 6 hours
c. Liquid 5 mg/5 mL; suppository 2.5, 5 mg
3. Metoclopramide (Reglan)
a. 10 mg IV/IM every 4 hours
b. 10 mg PO every 6 hours
c. Liquid, 5 mg/5 mL
4. Hydroxyzine (Vistaril)
a. 25 to 50 mg IM every 6 hours
b. 50 mg PO every 8 hours
5. Ondansetron (Zofran)
a. 4 mg IV every 4 to 6 hours (8 mg if severe)
b. 8 mg PO every 8 hours
c. Solution, 4 mg/5 mL
6. Scopolamine patch (Transderm Scōp), 1 disk (1.5 mg) every 3 days
a. 1 disk = 1.5 mg. Onset over 3 to 6 hours
7. Trimethobenzamide (Tigan)
a. 250 mg PO every 6 hours
b. Capsules 250 mg, suppository 100/200 mg

C. Anticonstipation agents
1. Bisacodyl (Dulcolax) 10 to 15 mg PO every 8 hours; 10 mg PR PRN
2. Docusate calcium (Surfak) 240 mg PO daily
3. Docusate sodium (Colace) 100 mg PO twice daily
4. Mg citrate 150 to 300 mL PO twice daily
5. Mg hydroxide (milk of magnesia) 30 to 60 mL PO every 8 hours
6. Docusate, casanthranol (Peri-Colace) 1 to 2 caplets PO at bedtime; 15 to 30 mL PO at bedtime
7. Polycarbophil (Fibercon) 1 g PO 4 times daily
8. Polyethylene glycol (MiraLax) 1 heaping tbsp (17 g) in 8 oz liquid daily
9. Psyllium (Metamucil) 1 tsp in liquid three times daily
10. Senna (Senokot) 2 tablets or 15 mL syrup three times daily
11. Senokot S (Senna + Docusate) 2 tablets PO daily

Note: *Typically combine a bulk and a motility agent.*

D. Pruritus
1. Diphenhydramine (Benadryl)
a. 12.5 to 50 mg IV every 8 hours
b. 25 to 50 mg PO every 8 hours
2. Hydroxyzine (Vistaril)
a. 25 to 50 mg IM every 8 hours
b. 50 mg PO every 8 hours
3. Naloxone infusion

a. 0.1 to 0.5 µg/kg/hr
b. Mix 1000 µg naloxone/250 mL normal saline (NS)
c. Titrate to lowest rate that decreases itching

E. Respiratory depression
1. Naloxone 100 to 200 µg IV
2. Infusion 0.5 to 5 µg/kg per hour (see above mix)

VI. PEARLS

A. Make the patient comfortable with bolus therapy before starting the PCA.

B. Frequently reassess.

C. Avoid meperidine.

D. Write for appropriate PRN and prophylactic adjuncts.

E. Consider opiate rotation if there is inadequate analgesia.

F. Think in terms of mg/kg or µg/kg, not fixed doses.

Alternative Routes and Methods of Drug Delivery

W. James Phillips

I. SUBCUTANEOUS (SC)

This route is typically chosen in the setting of chronic pain when nonparenteral approaches have become ineffective and in situations of difficult intravenous areas when parenteral titration and maintenance are required.

A. If SC delivery is employed, the following guidelines may be useful.
1. Use a 22-gauge Angiocath or butterfly needle placed in one of the following areas:
a. Over the deltoid muscle
b. Abdominal wall
c. Buttocks, iliac crest
d. Over the quadriceps muscle
2. Change sites every 48 to 72 hours to minimize infections.
3. The recommended maximum hourly infusion rate to avoid swelling is 2 to 5 mL/hr.
4. To minimize volume, maximize concentration; specialized preparations may be needed.
a. Fentanyl 50 µg/mL
b. Morphine 50 mg/mL
c. Hydromorphone 30–50 mg/mL

B. Pearls
1. SC dose = IV dose
2. May use PCA with SC administration

II. RECTAL

This route represents an alternative to oral dosing and potential avoidance of hepatic first-pass effects. About 50% of the administrated drug bypasses the liver. The rectal route is most often used for temporary or terminal care.

A. Oral administration may not be feasible in the presence of:
1. Nausea and vomiting
2. NPO status
3. Esophageal disease
4. Bowel obstruction
5. Malabsorption syndromes

B. Disadvantages of rectal administration include:
1. Variable systemic availability
2. Poor patient acceptance

3. Contraindicated in the presence of neutropenia or thrombocytopenia
4. Difficult in the presence of rectal mucosal disease or diarrhea

C. Dosage forms available
1. Aspirin: 120, 125, 300, 500 mg every 6 to 8 hours
2. Morphine suppositories: 5, 10, 20, 30 mg every 3 to 4 hours
3. Hydromorphone suppositories: 3 mg every 4 to 6 hours
4. Diazepam: 2.5, 5 mg, 15, 20 mg (twin packs), 10 mg
5. Indomethacin: 50 mg every 8 hours

D. Pearls
1. Immediate- and sustained-release oral tablets and solutions may be used rectally (ie, MS Contin)
2. Place past the rectal sphincter.

III. TRANSDERMAL DELIVERY

Fentanyl, lidocaine, capsaicin, and EMLA: The rate limiting step for any agent is the passive diffusion through the stratum corneum of the skin.

A. Fentanyl (Duragesic)
1. Fentanyl is the only commercially available opioid for this route of administration. The general maximum recommended dose is 300 µg/hr. Fentanyl is supplied as 25-, 50-, 75-, and 100-µg/hour patches. Wearing more than one patch at a time is acceptable if necessary for chronic analgesia.
2. Target plasma fentanyl levels are gradually reached over 12 to 18 hours, and likewise dissipate over 20 to 24 hours after the final patch is removed.
3. Advantages
a. Compliance
b. Ease of administration
c. Avoid first-first pass effect
d. Consistent analgesia
4. Disadvantages
a. Cost
b. Delayed respiratory depression
c. Inability to rapidly titrate
d. Less useful for acute or transitioning pain

B. Lidocaine 5% (Lidoderm)
1. Supplied as a 10 × 14-cm patch containing 700 mg lidocaine in an aqueous base. The mechanism of action is blockade or neuronal sodium channels. Clinically active abnormal sodium channels may play a role in both neuropathic pain states and in the cases of peripheral inflammation such as osteoarthritis. Lidocaine may also modulate the production of peripheral nitric oxide and release of inflammatory mediators.

2. The lidocaine patch is intended as a local treatment, in which the patch is placed over the site of maximal pain, that is, an arthritic knee or the foot in a case of peripheral neuropathy, or in the zone of innervation in postherpetic neuralgia.
3. U.S. Food and Drug Administration (FDA) recommendations are for up to 3 patches to be worn no longer than 12 hours in a 24-hour period. Clinical practice suggests that 18 hours on, 6 hours off may be acceptable. One to 2 weeks may be necessary to fully evaluate efficacy.

C. Capsaicin (Zostrix)

1. Capsaicin is a naturally occurring substance derived from the red chili pepper. It is available over the counter as a cream or lotion in strengths of 0.025% and 0.075%.
2. The mechanisms of action appear to be:
a. Substance P depletion from presynaptic terminals. This diminishes the function of some nociceptive fibers.
b. Reversible damage to underlying epidermal nerve fibers, that is, transient neurodegeneration.
3. Like lidocaine, capsaicin is intended for application directly over the site of inflammation or neuropathic pain. Peripheral neuropathy, scar pain, and joint inflammation are some of the acceptable indications.
4. Topical capsaicin is generally applied 3 to 4 times daily. The area of application should not be washed for 1 hour afterward. Analgesia usually takes 2 to 6 weeks of daily use.
5. A transient burning sensation occurs after application for the first 3 to 10 days. This limits compliance. Wash hands after use and avoid exposure to broken skin, eyes, mucous membranes, and genitalia.

D. Eutectic mixture of local anesthetic (EMLA)

1. This is a cream consisting of lidocaine 2.5% and prilocaine 2.5% applied to skin under an occlusive dressing. It is intended for use on intact skin only. EMLA anesthetizes the underlying skin by topical anesthetic actions, that is, sodium channel blockade. Skin anesthesia peaks over 2 to 3 hours and lasts for 1 to 2 hours after removal. Beware systemic uptake if left longer than 3 hours. Typical side effects are minor and may include:
a. Skin pallor
b. Redness
c. Pruritus
d. Rash
2. Beware the rare risk for prilocaine and associated methemoglobinemia.
3. Indications
a. Skin anesthesia for venipuncture or IV insertion.
b. Painful neuropathy
c. Postsurgical scar pain—acute and chronic
4. Dose: apply 2.5 g or 1 disk to area at least 1 hour before procedure.

IV. TRANSMUCOSAL

A. This typically refers to both oral and nasal routes of administration.

B. Nasal: the nasal mucosa offers a surface area similar to that of the mouth. This system bypasses hepatic first-pass effects. Two to three drops will cover most of the nasal passage. Higher volumes are swallowed.

1. Butorphanol
a. This is the only commercially available analgesic nasal spray (Stadol NS. Dose: 1 spray = 1 mg in 1 nostril every 3 to 4 hours).
b. Like all mixed agonist-antagonists, this agent has a ceiling effect and may counteract the effect of pure agents.
c. Onset of analgesia is 15 minutes, with peak effects in 30 to 60 minutes.
2. Fentanyl, morphine, and midazolam have been used intranasally. Fentanyl in particular has a high bioavailability.
a. Fentanyl: 50 µg/mL
   (1) Dose: 2 to 3 µg/kg intranasally
   (2) Minimal irritation
b. Morphine: 20 mg/mL or 2mg/gtt
   (1) Dose: 10 to 20 mg
   (2) Expect some degree of mucosal irritation with morphine.
c. Midazolam: 5 mg/mL
   (1) Dose: 0.25 mg/kg for preprocedural sedation

C. Lozenges
1. Fentanyl (Actiq) lollipops
a. Available as 200-, 400-, 600-, 800-, 1200-, and 1600-µg lozenges.
b. Maximum recommended is 4 per day.
c. This agent is generally recommended for immediate sedation or breakthrough pain.
d. Beware high plasma levels and risk for respiratory depression.
2. Fentanyl buccal lozenges are also available (Fentora).
a. Exhibit a 10–15 minute onset
b. Only re-dose after 30 minutes
c. Buccal lozenge dose is 25–30% of the oral lollipop dose!
d. Available as 100, 200, and 400 µg tablets.

Note: *Do NOT bite lozenges—higher plasma levels may occur.*

D. Buccal or sublingual
Buccal or sublingual administration of oral tablets (eg, morphine) involves placing the tablet in the buccal space above the gingival line for gradual absorption. Sublingual administration of opioid solutions such as morphine (20 mg/mL) or hydromorphone (1 mg/mL) a few drops at a

time may be successful. Incremental administration of a few drops at a time minimizes the amount of drug that is swallowed.

V. INHALED AND NEBULIZED DELIVERY

Aerosol delivery of morphine sulfate has been described primarily for relieving dyspnea in terminal cancer patients. The technique is to nebulize the agent in exactly the same fashion as if administering a β agonist for asthma.

A. Our protocol is 10 to 20 mg (roughly 0.25 to 0.3 mg/kg) morphine sulfate in 4 mL total volume repeated every 2 to 4 hours.

B. Mucosal irritation or cough is nearly nonexistent.

C. This is a useful technique for:

1. Cases of difficult intravenous access (sickle cell pain crises)
2. Preparation for fiberoptic bronchoscopy when combined with nebulized lidocaine (anecdotal)

VI. INTRATHECAL AND EPIDURAL ADMINISTRATION

See Chapter 10 for a more complete review. These routes are options of either last resort for chronic pain syndromes or planned interventions in the case of postoperative or postinjury states. A variety of agents have been used by both single-shot and catheter-based infusion techniques by anesthesiologists.

A. These routes are considered when:
1. Other routes have reached maximum effective dosing levels.
2. Intolerable side effects preclude further dose escalation.
3. A particularly difficult pain syndrome is encountered.

B. Advantages include:
1. Lower doses (1:100) compared with IV
2. Prolonged duration of action (18 to 24 hours for intrathecal morphine)
3. Fewer systemic side effects

C. Disadvantages include delayed respiratory effects (24 hours)
This is more common with hydrophilic (morphine) than with lipophilic opioids (fentanyl), which rapidly absorbs into local neural tissue close to the site of injection rather than having a tendency to spread to central respiratory centers through cerebrospinal fluid.

D. Potential central axis agents may include the following:
1. Opioids: morphine is the only FDA-approved opiate for intrathecal use. Doses are 5 to 15 µg/kg, depending on opioid naivety. Morphine is

also available as a lipid encapsulated depot preparation for single-shot epidural placement with analgesia possible for 24 to 48 hours (Depodur). Other opioids that have been used intrathecally or epidurally include hydromorphone, fentanyl, sufentanil, and methadone.

2. Local anesthetics: used epidurally in preservative-free form to provide sensory analgesia in low enough concentration to spare motor function. Sympathetic blockade is typical, even with low concentration.

3. α Agonists: clonidine is FDA approved for epidural use as an analgesic adjuvant by infusion. Because it is an antihypertensive, drops in blood pressure and heart rate may occur in a dose-related fashion. It has an opiate-sparing effect and may be used to alleviate opiate withdrawal symptoms.

4. γ-Aminobutyric acid (GABA)-A agonist: midazolam has been used as a spinal cord analgesic (small case series).

5. N-methyl-D-aspartate receptor antagonist: ketamine has been used epidurally to complement epidural analgesia for acute and chronic pain. Psychomimetic side effects and lack of preservative-free preparations are limitations.

6. GABA-B Agonist: baclofen is FDA approved for intrathecal infusion for spasticity syndromes. It has analgesic potential in some neuropathic pain states.

7. N-type calcium channel blocker: PRIALT, formerly SNX-111 or ziconotide, is a calcium channel blocker derived from snail venom. It has potential neuropathic analgesic for central axis utilization. Calcium channel influx at the dorsal horn is affected.

E. Clinical pearls

1. All central axis agents should be preservative free. The agents themselves are rarely neurotoxic.

2. Hydrophilic agents spread rostrally. Lipophilic agents are more likely to provide dermatomal analgesia.

3. Epidural opiates work by diffusion across the dura to the dorsal horn and nerve roots.

4. Meperidine has local anesthetic activity and may cause motor blockade epidurally.

Intrathecal and Epidural Analgesia

W. James Phillips and Anna Lerant

10

I. AN OVERVIEW OF CENTRAL AXIS (SPINAL CORD) PHARMACOLOGY

A. Proper drug utilization necessitates a clear understanding of receptor types and actions and interactions.

B. This discussion is intended as a broad overview so that the reader may understand where the many available agents fit into the larger scheme of spinal analgesia.

C. Potential receptor types and mechanisms available for dorsal horn pain signal modulation include (Fig. 10-1, Table 10-1):

1. Sodium (Na) channel blockade
2. Opioid
3. Monoamine
4. Excitatory amino acids (EAA)
5. Inhibitory amino acids (IAA)
6. Calcium channel blockade
7. Cholinergic
8. Purine
9. Somatostatin

D. Sodium channel blockade

This is the nonspecific and broad neuronal conduction block that occurs with the intrathecal and epidural local anesthetics in the same fashion as if a peripheral nerve is blocked.

E. Opioids

1. The spinal cord dorsal horn contains mu (μ), kappa (κ), and delta (δ) opioid receptors. Presynaptic opioid effect is to decrease the release of excitatory neurotransmitters such as substance P (SP). The postsynaptic action functionally serves to decrease the excitability of dorsal horn neurons. These effects are at least partially mediated by potassium channel modulation.
2. Opioids that have been used intrathecally and epidurally, in more or less decreasing order of frequency, include:
a. Morphine (only one approved by the U.S. Food and Drug Administration [FDA] for spinal use)
b. Fentanyl
c. Hydromorphone
d. Meperidine

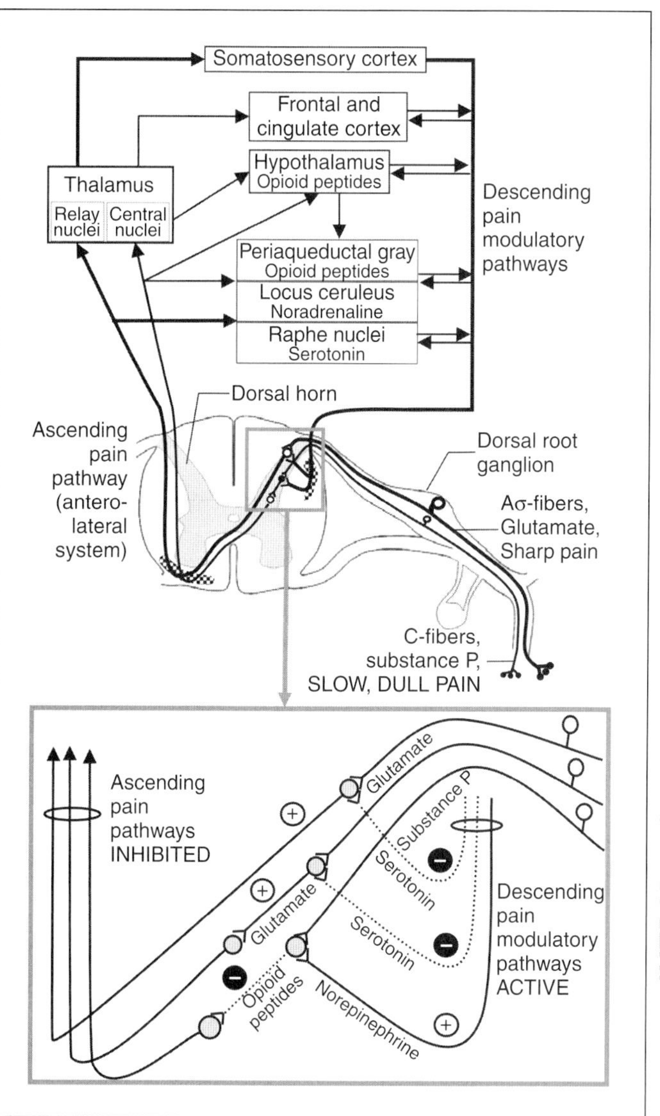

FIG. 10-1

Pain pathways and the anatomy of the dorsal horn of the spinal cord.

TABLE 10-1

NEUROTRANSMITTERS AND PHARMACOLOGIC TARGETS AT THE DORSAL HORN OF THE SPINAL CORD

	Primary Sensory Neuron	Interneuron	Descending Modulatory Pathway	Ascending Pain Sensory Pathway
Neurotransmitters and their receptors	*Substance P NK1 receptor*	*Glutamate NMDA receptor* *Aspartate NMDA receptor* *Ca^{++} channel* **Opiates: κ, μ receptors** **GABA: GABA-A receptor** **Glycine: Gly receptor**	**Serotonin (5HT-2 receptor, serotonin transporter)** **Norepinephrine (α_1 and α_2-adrenergic receptors, norepinephrine transporter)** **Opiates: κ, μ receptors**	*Glutamate NMDA receptor*
Enzymes		*Cyclooxygenase* Nitric oxide synthase (NOS)		

Italics indicate that the drug's inhibitors or antagonists promote anesthesia; boldface indicates that the drug's agonists or increased activity promote anesthesia.

e. Methadone
f. Sufentanil
g. Alfentanil
h. Buprenorphine

F. Monoamines
1. α_2 Agonists: This is a postsynaptic dorsal horn receptor that inhibits pain impulses. NO β effects have been demonstrated.
2. Examples:
a. Clonidine: a selective α_2 agonist produces analgesia through nonopioid mechanisms after intrathecal or epidural administration. It potentiates the analgesic effect of both central axis opioids and local anesthetics. Dexmedetomidine is another selective α_2 agonist used intravenously.
b. Epinephrine: when added to intrathecal or epidural local anesthetic, it not only prolongs the duration but also **increases the quality** of the block.
c. Tricyclic antidepressants: have part of their antinociceptive effect mediated through blockage of norepinephrine reuptake at the spinal cord with enhanced α_2 agonist action.
d. Serotonin (5-HT) modulation also produces an analgesic effect because $5\text{-}HT_2$ receptors are antinociceptive.

G. Excitatory amino acids (EAAs)
1. Aspartate and glutamate are the primary examples. Receptors for these excitatory neurotransmitters are located not only on the spinal cord dorsal horn but also in peripheral nerves and the dorsal root ganglia. The primary EAA receptor at the dorsal horn is the *N*-methyl-D-aspartate (NMDA) receptor. Activation of this receptor produces a state of facilitated central pain processing, that is, a sensitized spinal cord.
2. NMDA receptor blockades include:
a. Ketamine
b. Dextromethorphan
c. Methadone (unique effect among opioids)
d. Magnesium
3. Example: Ketamine is the only one of these with some track record of use as an *epidurally* administered analgesic with single-dose duration of 3 to 4 hours. Ketamine also modulates dorsal horn adrenergic, cholinergic, and 5-HT receptors. Side effects have included hypertension, tachycardia, sedation, and dysphoria.

H. Inhibitory amino acids
1. γ-Aminobutyric acid (GABA) and glycine are the primary examples.
2. GABA-A receptor: modulated by alcohol, barbiturates, and benzodiazepines (oral diazepam for back pain and spasm likely exerts its antispasm effect here. Example: Midazolam has been used intrathecally acutely for postoperative pain and chronically for a variety of musculoskeletal pain syndromes.

3. GABA-B receptor: Baclofen is a relatively selective GABA-B agonist. Example: Baclofen has been used fairly widely through a chronic intrathecal infusion system for cerebral palsy and multiple sclerosis–related spasticity. It may also have an actual analgesic effect.

I. Calcium channel blockade

1. Calcium channel function is an important part of neuronal excitability. Of the several calcium channel subtypes, the L and N types may offer antinociceptive potential.
2. Example:
a. L-type channels: modulated by traditional calcium modulators such as verapamil, which has been used epidurally
b. N-type channels: ziconotide is an FDA-approved agent for intrathecal use in patients with pain refractory to systemic modalities or intrathecal morphine. Severe psychological dysfunction has been reported with its use.

J. Cholinergic

Acetylcholinesterase inhibitors (which increase central level of acetylcholine) produce an antinociceptive effect. Example: Neostigmine has been used intrathecally with moderate analgesia but with limitations of gastrointestinal side effects and the same degree of lower extremity paresis.

K. Purine receptors

There are three purine receptor subtypes (A_1, A_2, A_3) at the dorsal horn. Example: Adenosine has been used intravenously to address neuropathic pain, and animal data suggest that intrathecal A_1 agonists exert an antinociceptive effect.

L. Somatostatin

Receptors likely inhabit not only the spinal cord but also the brainstem centers. Example: Octreotide, a somatostatin analogue, has been used intrathecally as a chronic infusion for nonmalignant pain.

Note: *These examples illustrate the large and ever-expanding avenues for pain modulation at the spinal cord level. The reader is referred to in-depth texts for a more extensive review.*

II. PRACTICAL ASPECTS OF INTRATHECAL ANALGESIA

A. Intrathecal anatomy and needle placement are shown in Figure 10-2.

B. The main agents for intrathecal analgesia techniques are the opioids. A key property to understand when choosing a drug is hydrophilicity versus lipophilicity. Lipophilic agents such as fentanyl are rapidly absorbed into neural tissue or blood vessels and migrate minimally cephalad in the cerebrospinal fluid (CSF).

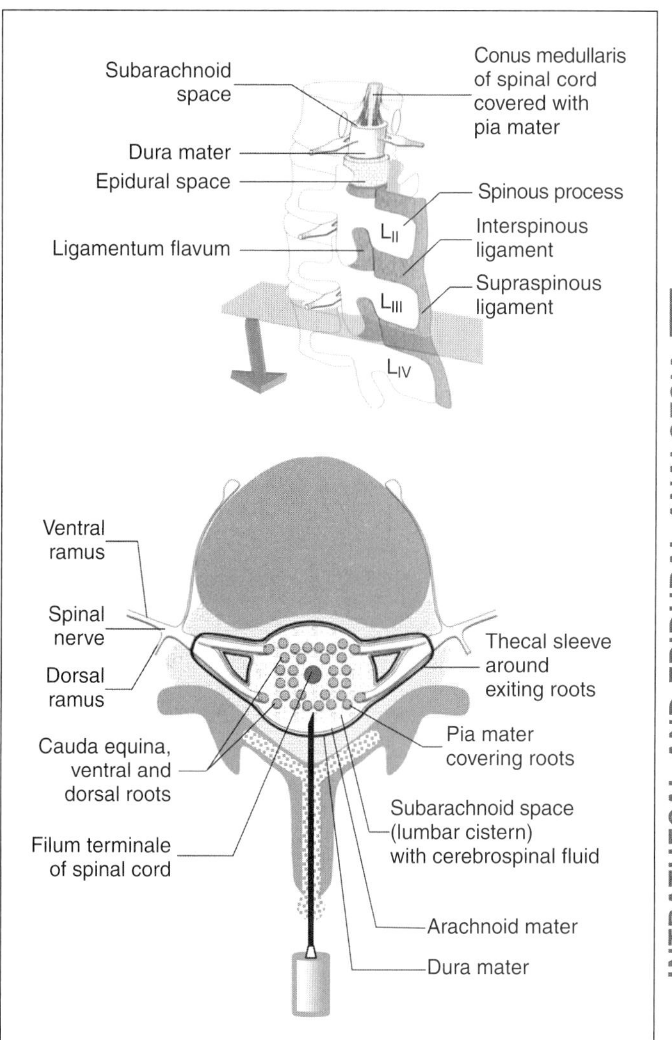

FIG. 10-2

Intrathecal (subarachnoid) anatomy and needle placement.

C. Hydrophilic agents such as morphine and hydromorphone migrate cephalad in the CSF and exert analgesic action at higher dermatomes. Lack of uptake into the bloodstream markedly prolongs the duration of action. Higher doses produce more cephalad migration, more analgesia at higher dermatomes, and greater incidence of respiratory depression and nausea and vomiting due to brainstem effects.

D. Practically speaking, the lipophilic agents do not last long enough, and preservative-free morphine is the mainstay of intrathecal analgesic techniques.

1. Onset of action is about 1 hour, with dose-dependent duration of 6 to 24 hours after typical lumbar placement. Uses may include:
a. Postoperative pain after lower extremity, abdominal, or thoracic surgery. Beware that respiratory depression is additive with parenterally administered sedatives and analgesics and in the presence of significant preexisting comorbidities.
b. "Single-shot" (e.g., non-catheter delivered) use for hospitalized severe pain flares such as advanced cancer pain, nonoperative treatment of extremity injuries, and so forth.
c. Single-shot for labor analgesia
2. Lumbar single-shot intrathecal doses
a. Doses are given in Table 10-2.
b. Lower doses should be considered for elderly and chronically ill patients. Delayed respiratory depressions may be seen even with the lower dose ranges.
3. Side effects
a. Respiratory depression is a risk for up to 24 hours after administration. Naloxone standing orders typically accompany intrathecal opiate orders.
b. Nausea and vomiting may occur in up to 30% of cases after intrathecal or epidural opioids. This is likely due to cephalad migration and action at central and brainstem vomiting centers (area postrema).
c. Pruritus may be the most common side effect after central axis opiates. It may occur in any distribution and is a NEUROGENIC and not an allergic event. It is associated with all opiates and likely involves an opiate-trigeminal nucleus effect. Because it is a receptor-mediated phenomenon,

TABLE 10-2

LUMBAR SINGLE-SHOT INTRATHECAL DOSES

	Morphine	Fentanyl	Sufentanil
Lower extremity pain, lower abdominal pain	0.1–0.2 mg	5–25 μg	2–10 μg
Upper abdominal pain (eg, postoperative)	0.2–0.4 mg	Not enough spread	
Thoracic pain (eg, postoperative)	0.4–0.7 mg	Not enough spread	

tolerance often develops after 1 or 2 days. Treatment is symptomatic with antihistamines, and rarely, very-low-dose naloxone infusions (naloxone, 1 mg/250 mL 9% saline infused at 0.5 to 1 µg/kg per hour).
  d. Urinary retention is also an opioid receptor–mediated phenomenon through sacral neurons. The incidence is difficult to ascertain because postoperative and postinjury urinary retention may be multifactorial. Bladder catheterization may be needed, or a low-dose naloxone infusion as outlined previously.

E. Intrathecal opioid caveats
1. Hydrophilic agents such as morphine produce higher-level and longer-lasting analgesia, but at the expense of a higher incidence of side effects.
2. Respiratory depression may occur up to 24 hours after intrathecal morphine, and the incidence increases in elderly and infirm patients and with co-administration of other sedative-hypnotics.
3. Particular attention must be paid to the *transition* to oral or intravenous (ie, patient-controlled analgesia [PCA]) analgesics as the effect of the spinal opiate wanes. The need for analgesia and the risk for respiratory depression must be carefully *and* repetitively monitored.

III. PRACTICAL ASPECTS OF EPIDURAL ANALGESIA
A. Epidural anatomy and needle placement are shown in Figure 10-3.

B. The advantages of epidural over intrathecal delivery of analgesics include:
1. More amenable to continuous catheter-based delivery.
2. Ability to provide segmental or dermatomal analgesia.
3. Lower incidence of hypotension, respiratory depression, and headache.
4. More amenable to utilization of drug combinations (usually low-dose local anesthetic and opioid).
5. Catheters may remain in place 3 to 5 days until other analgesic methods are in effect.
6. Onset of sympathectomy or hypotension is more gradual owing to the need for diffusion across the dura.
7. Onset of analgesia will likewise be more gradual.
8. No INITIAL effect of hydrophilicity versus lipophilicity on drug migration or diffusion

C. Typical catheter placement sites in relation to injury or incision location are given in Table 10-3.

D. Drug choice
1. Typical agents are local anesthetics and opioids. The best analgesia is when both are used as a combination infusion and both dorsal horn

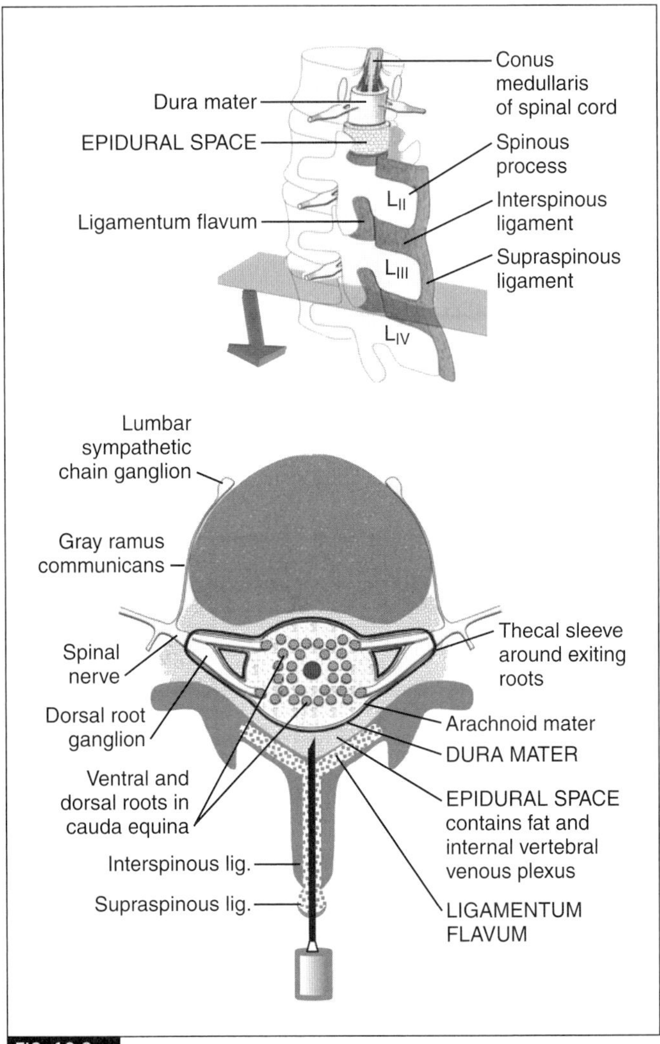

FIG. 10-3

Epidural anatomy and needle placement.

TABLE 10-3

CATHETER PLACEMENT SITES IN RELATION TO INJURY OR INCISION LOCATION

Incision or Injury Site	Examples	Vertebral Catheter Placement
Thoracic	Thoracotomy	T4–T8
	Rib fracture pain	
Upper abdominal	Exploratory laparotomy	T6–T10
	Pancreatic pain	
Flank, renal	Nephrectomy	T8–T10
	Renal colic	
Lower abdominal	Cesarean birth	T8–T12
	Prostatectomy	
Lower extremity	Hip surgery	L1–L4
	Femur fracture	

opiate agonist action and spinal nerve root conduction modulation (local anesthetic) produce a synergistic effect (Table 10-4).

2. By combining the two classes, *at lower doses*, the DISADVANTAGES of each may be minimized:

a. Local anesthetic disadvantages:

(1) Motor block

(2) Hypotension

(3) Urinary retention

b. Opioid disadvantages:

(1) Respiratory depression

(2) Pruritus

(3) Urinary retention

(4) Nausea and vomiting

3. Typical local anesthetics used are BUPIVACAINE and ROPIVACAINE because of their tendency to provide a preferential analgesia with *less motor block*.

4. Typical opiates used are morphine, hydromorphone, and fentanyl. With the highly lipophilic agents such as fentanyl, most of the analgesia is due to systemic uptake and the authors see *NO* advantage to using these agents epidurally.

5. The *added* advantage of epidural morphine (hydrophilic) is that it will diffuse into the CSF and migrate (slowly) cephalad and may give higher dermatomal analgesia even with a lumbar catheter.

E. Catheter site choice

1. Thoracic epidural catheter advantages

a. Congruent and dermatomal analgesia ("segmental")

b. Potential sparing of lumbar and sacral roots

(1) Less urinary retention

(2) Less lower extremity motor block

TABLE 10-4

USEFUL STARTING EPIDURAL DRUG CHOICES AND COMBINATIONS

Catheter Location	Pain Site	Local Anesthetic	Opioid	Infusion Rate
Thoracic*	Congruent	Ropivacaine 0.1%, *or* Bupivacaine 0.125%	Morphine 40–80 µg/mL Hydromorphone 5–40 µg/mL Fentanyl 2–5 µg/mL	5–8 mL/hr
Lumbar	Congruent (pelvis, lower extremity)	Same	Same	6–10 mL/hr
Lumbar	Noncongruent (thoracic)	0	Morphine 40–80 µg/mL	Same

*Reduce infusion rate 30% in elderly patients.

c. Lower drug requirements (reduce by one third from lumbar)
d. Dermatomal volume = 1 mL/dermatome
2. Lumbar catheter advantages
a. Technically easier
b. Good for pelvic and lower extremity surgery
c. Dermatomal volumes =1.5 mL/dermatome

F. Epidural morphine caveats
1. Total drug infusion 50 to 300 µg/hour
2. Onset time after bolus = 1 to 2 hours
3. Epidural morphine loading doses are shown in Table 10-5.

G. Additives to epidural solution
1. Epinephrine may improve analgesia and sensory block. Typically included at a concentration of 2 to 5 µg/mL. Acts at spinal α_2 receptors.
2. Clonidine (Duraclon) also acts at spinal α_2 receptors. The enhanced analgesia is partially offset by the potential side effects of sedation, hypotension, and bradycardia.

Note: *Epidural morphine is also available as a single-shot depot preparation:* **DepoDur**. *This liposomal encapsulated preparation may be delivered as a single dose of 10 to 20 mg in 0.9% saline in the lumbar epidural space. After an onset time of 2 to 6 hours, analgesia may be experienced for up to 24 to 30 hours. The disadvantage of this agent is that overshoot or undershoot of analgesia does not allow dose titration. The main advantage is the lack of a catheter and enhanced patient mobility and possible decreased pharmacy drug infusion preparation costs.*

3. Dosage recommendations for the perioperative period are:
a. Cesarean birth: 10 mg
b. Lower extremity orthopedic surgery: 15 mg
c. Lower abdominal or pelvic surgery: 10 to 15 mg

H. Patient-controlled epidural analgesia (PCEA)
1. Just as a patient may self-administer intravenous (PCA) analgesics, epidural infusions may be programmed to offer a PCEA function.

TABLE 10-5

EPIDURAL MORPHINE LOADING DOSES

Age (yr)	Dose
15–44	4–6 mg
45–65	3 mg
65–75	2 mg
>75	1 mg

2. When the typical local anesthetic and opioid combination is used, the PCEA function and limits are typically calculated based on the opioid. Typical settings are given in Table 10-6.

I. Epidural pitfalls

1. Inadequate assessment or reassessment.
2. Failure to bolus or achieve analgesia before initiating an infusion (same as PCA).
3. Respiratory depression from the opiates. Beware sedative co-administration!
4. Hypotension or orthostasis from the local anesthetic (particularly if patient ambulating).
5. Not tailoring the drug to the patient and the specific medical conditions.
6. Forgetting contraindications and dangers such as low platelets, use of Coumadin, heparin, Lovenox, and similar drugs.

TABLE 10-6

TYPICAL **PCEA** SETTINGS

Drug	Bolus	Lockout	4-Hour Limit	Infusion
Morphine	40–100 µg	30–45 min	Infusion + 150 µg	100–300 µg/hr
Hydromorphone	5–10 µg	30–45 min	Infusion + 25 µg	10–40 µg/hr
Fentanyl	15–20 µg	10 min	Infusion + 1–2 µg/kg	0.5 µg/kg/hr

Common Nerve Blocks

Anna Lerant and W. James Phillips

I. OVERVIEW OF NERVE BLOCKS AND LOCAL ANESTHETIC USE

Successful neural blockade requires a detailed knowledge of surface landmarks and neural innervation, dermatomal and sclerotomal anatomy, and local anesthetic physiology and pharmacology. In the acute setting, peripheral nerve blocks may provide outstanding analgesia and also serve as a means to supplement the effects of parenteral sedatives and analgesics. Examples include femoral nerve blockade for femur fractures, cervical plexus blockade for analgesia for central venous access placement, and ankle blocks for foot procedures.

Nerve blocks that have been chosen for discussion here are those that may be performed utilizing surface landmark anatomy and an infiltration-type technique. Discussion of peripheral nerve stimulators, transarterial techniques, and so forth is beyond the scope of this chapter.

Peripheral nerve blocks anesthetize mixed peripheral nerves and produce anesthesia and skeletal muscle relaxation starting a few centimeters distal to the site of injection. Local anesthetics are intrinsic vasodilators, thus enhancing blood flow and their own redistribution. The addition of epinephrine, typically in a concentration of 5 µg/mL, offsets this effect and prolongs the duration of the block. Addition of epinephrine also decreases the peak blood concentration of a local anesthetic by 20% to 30%, thus offering some additional margin of safety.

Local anesthetic choices are generally lidocaine, mepivacaine, bupivacaine, and ropivacaine. The choice of these agents depends on desired duration, with lidocaine and mepivacaine providing 1 to 2 hours (depending on local blood flow and utilization of epinephrine) and bupivacaine providing 3 to 18 hours of effect, with longer durations from the inclusion of epinephrine.

Ropivacaine is of interest because it is a homologue of mepivacaine and bupivacaine and also is provided as a single levo-isomer rather than a racemic mixture like traditional agents. It is as protein bound as bupivacaine (also long lasting), but less lipid soluble, so it provides less motor block. Duration of effect from ropivacaine is modestly shorter than that from bupivacaine.

The availability of a single isomer drug is important because typically one of a drug's single isomers may contribute more to toxicity. A perfect example is bupivacaine, for which the dextro isomer causes most of the potentially profound cardiotoxic effects. Levo-bupivacaine is available outside of North America.

Proper drug utilization begins with understanding maximal acceptable dosing (fortunately not usually an issue with one or even two peripheral nerve blocks) and meticulous attention to frequent negative aspiration checks during the injection process. Most peripheral nerves course in proximity to blood vessels, so intravascular injection with local anesthetic toxicity must be avoided.

A. Useful peripheral nerve block concentrations are:
1. Lidocaine 1% to 1.5%
2. Mepivacaine 1% to 2%
3. Bupivacaine 0.25% to 0.5%
4. Ropivacaine 0.5% to 0.75%
5. Remember: "percent" $\times$ 10 = mg/mL (Example: 1% lidocaine = 1 $\times$ 10 = 10 mg/mL)

B. Maximum doses
1. Maximum doses without epinephrine
a. Lidocaine 4 mg/kg
b. Mepivacaine 7 mg/kg
c. Bupivacaine 2 mg/kg
d. Ropivacaine 3 mg/kg
2. With epinephrine 5 µg/mL, total dose may be increased by 30%—though be quite careful with bupivacaine!
a. Lidocaine 6 to 7 mg/kg
b. Mepivacaine 9 mg/kg
c. Bupivacaine 3 mg/kg
d. Ropivacaine—no epi effect

C. Most single peripheral nerve blocks require 5 to 8 mL for adequate blockade.
1. This assumes proper drug volume and concentration!
2. Onset is generally within 15 to 20 minutes.
3. The exception is femoral nerve block, which requires 12 to 15 mL for a solid block.

D. Typically, 22-gauge needles are chosen for peripheral nerve blocks. If available, "b" beveled needles (less sharp = more blunt) are chosen to minimize potential nerve trauma.
1. By carefully approaching the nerve site while simultaneously slowly injecting the agent, nerve injury and excessive discomfort can almost always be avoided.
2. Never inject while the patient is feeling a paresthesia; immediately stop needle motion, withdraw the needle slightly, and wait for the paresthesia to resolve before gently redirecting and continuing.
3. Example:
a. 70-kg patient with femur fracture for **femoral nerve block**
b. Longer analgesia is needed.
c. Bupivacaine maximum dose = 70 kg $\times$ 2 mg/kg = 140 mg; with epinephrine = 70 kg $\times$ 3 mg/kg = 210 mg

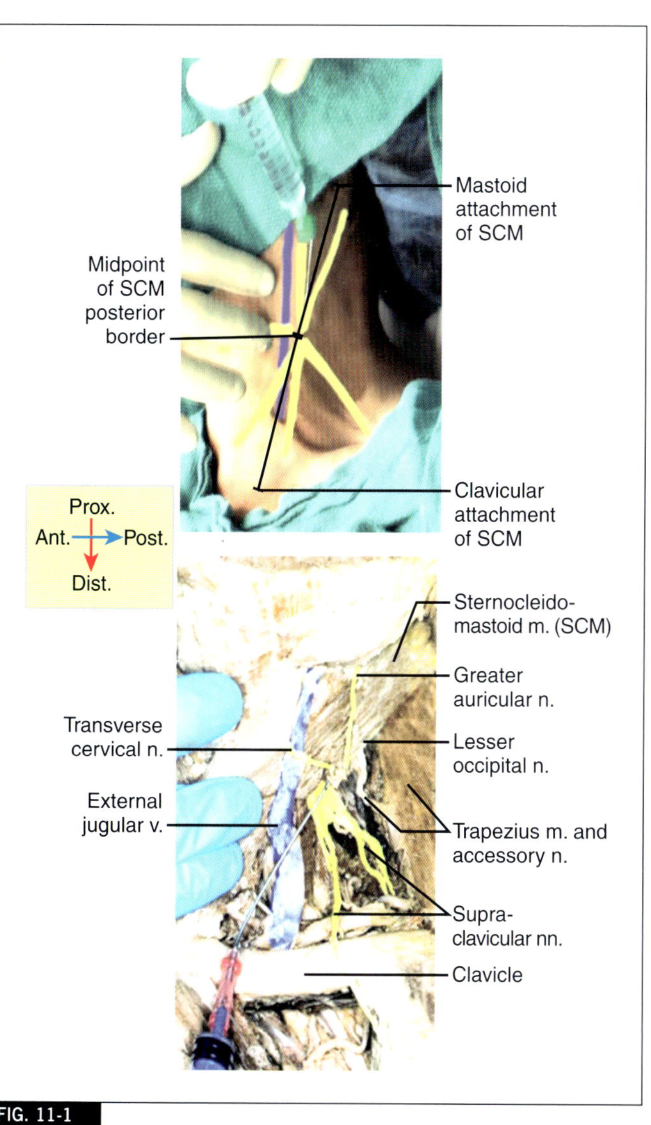

FIG. 11-1

Neck, left side, superficial cervical plexus block.

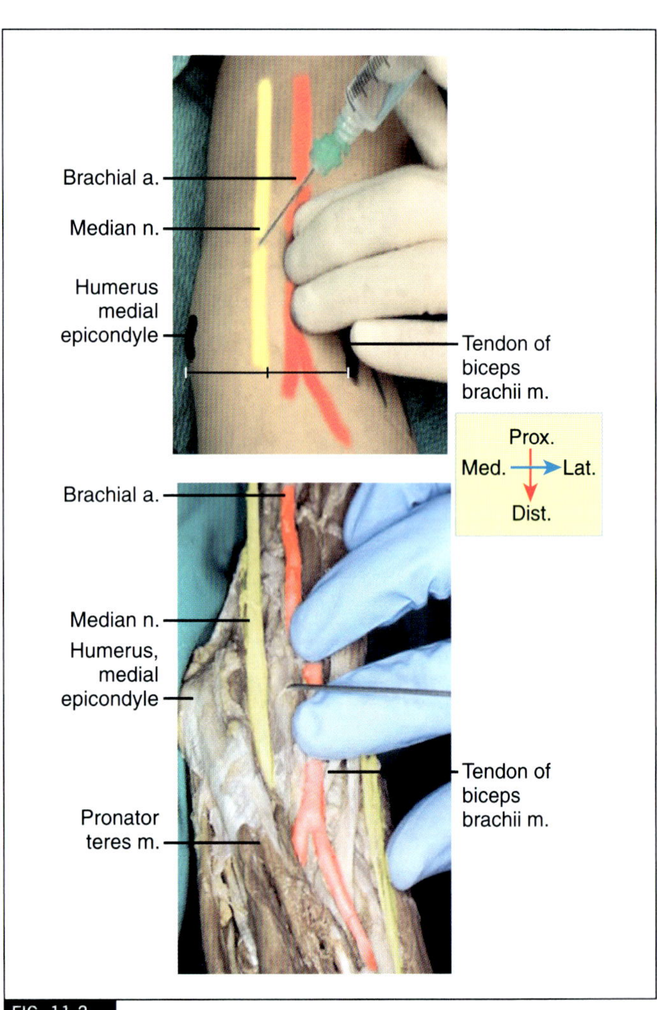

FIG. 11-2

Left elbow, median nerve block.

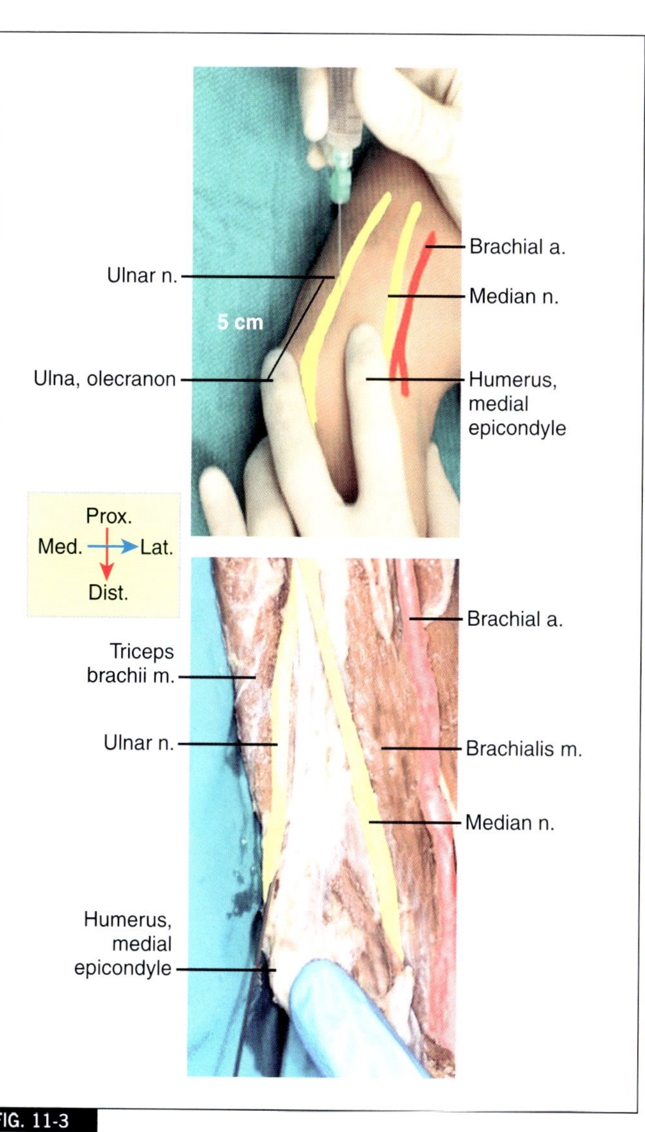

FIG. 11-3

Left elbow, ulnar nerve block.

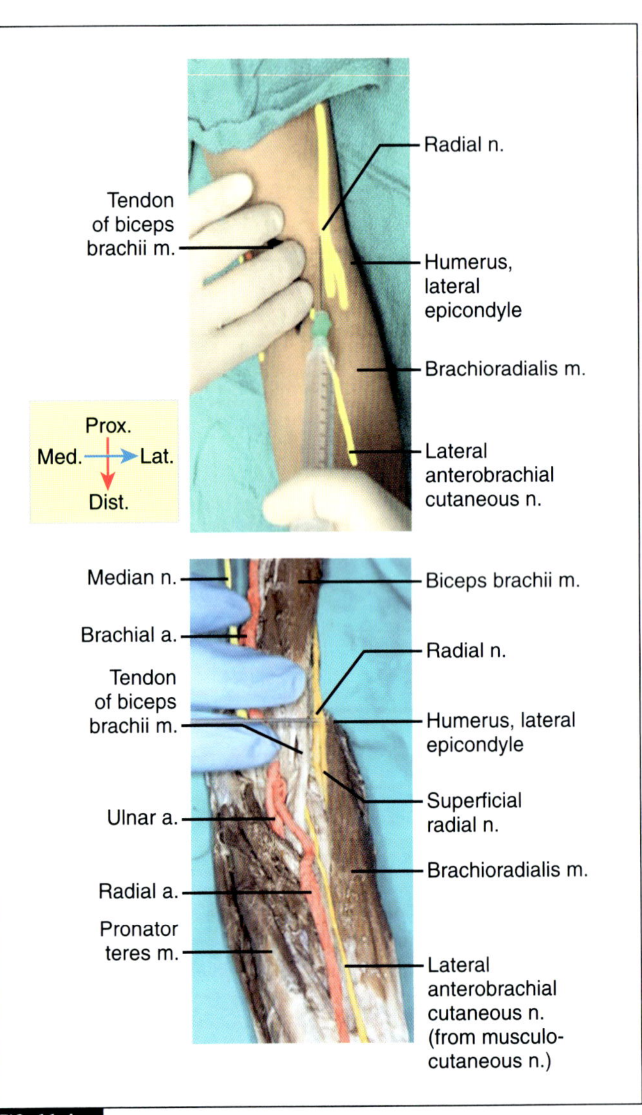

FIG. 11-4

Left elbow, radial nerve block.

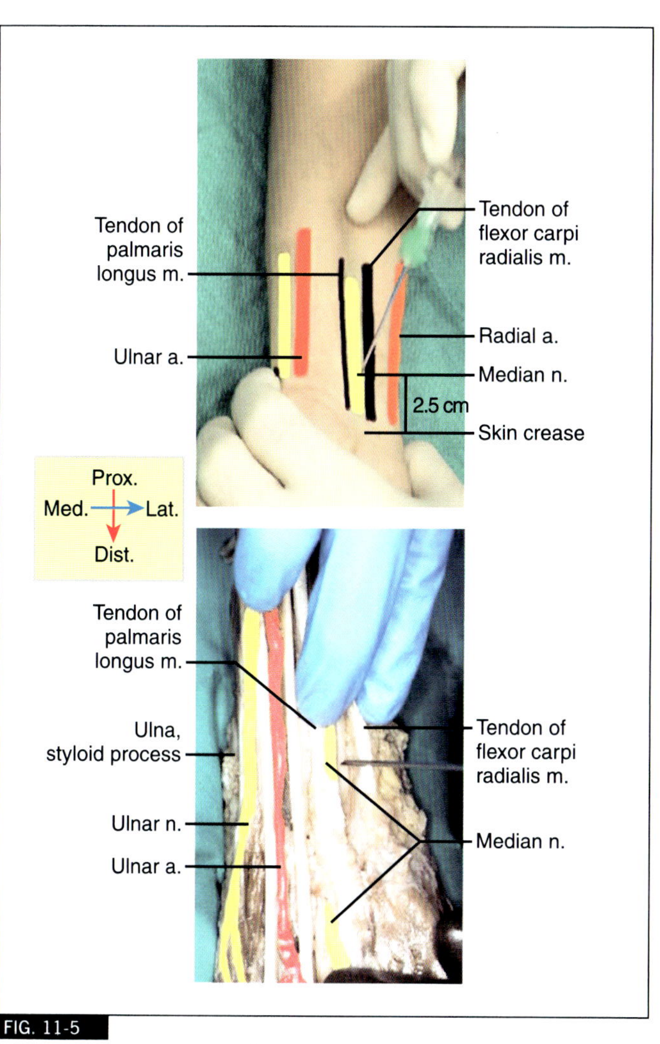

FIG. 11-5

Left wrist, forearm supinated, median nerve block.

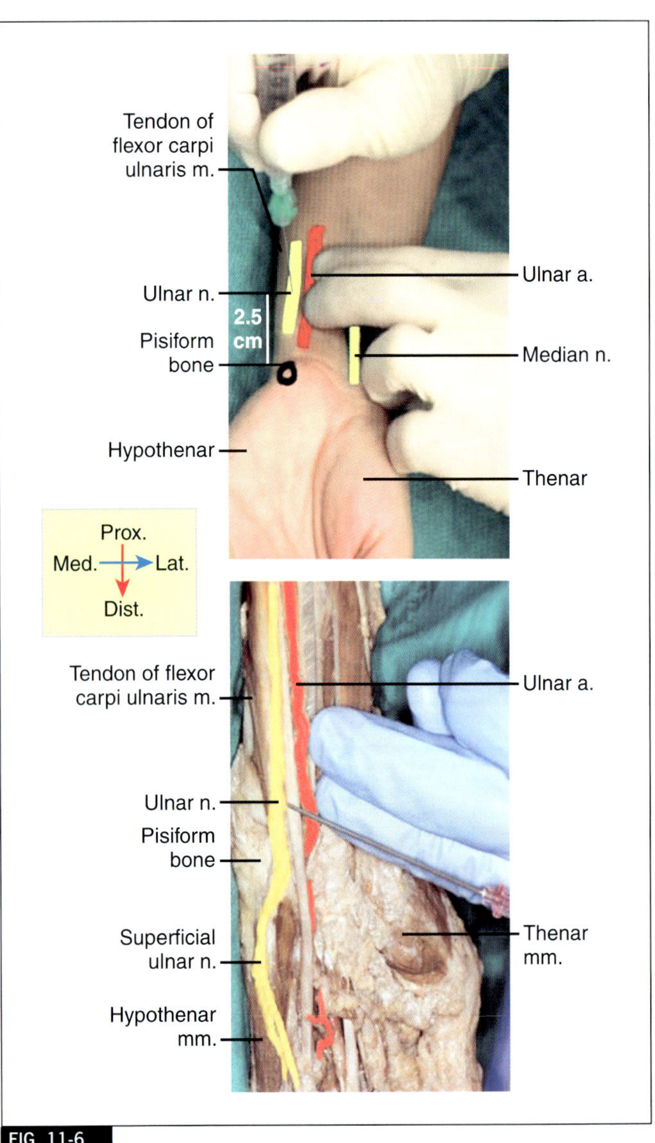

FIG. 11-6

Left wrist, forearm supinated, ulnar nerve block.

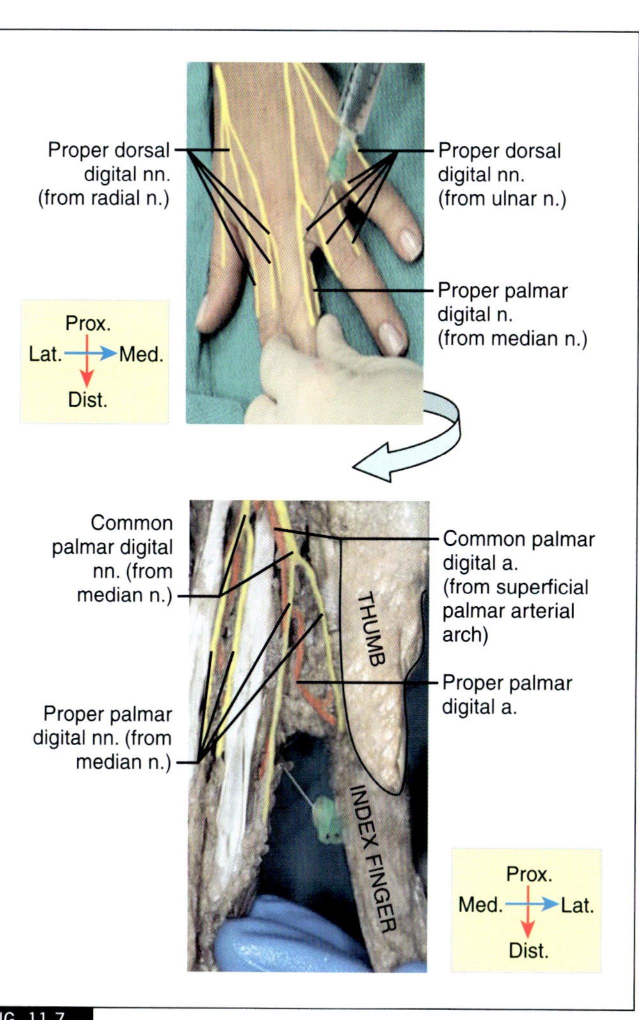

FIG. 11-7

Left hand, digital nerve block of middle finger. *Upper image*, Forearm pronated, dorsal view. *Lower image*, Forearm supinated, palmar (volar) view.

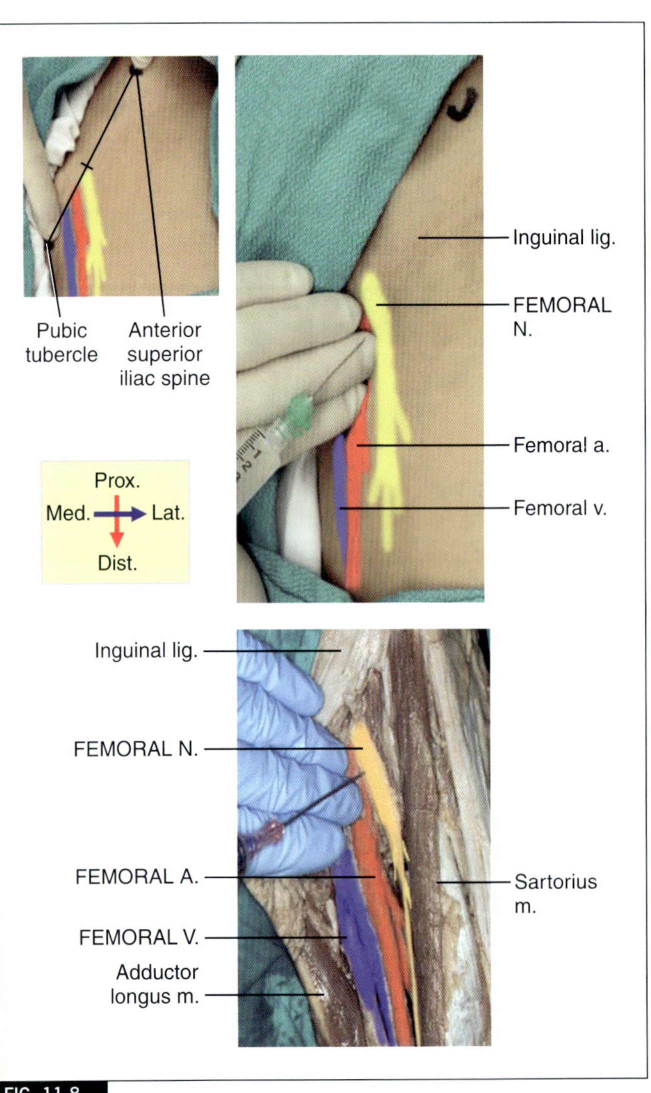

FIG. 11-8

Left femoral triangle, femoral nerve block.

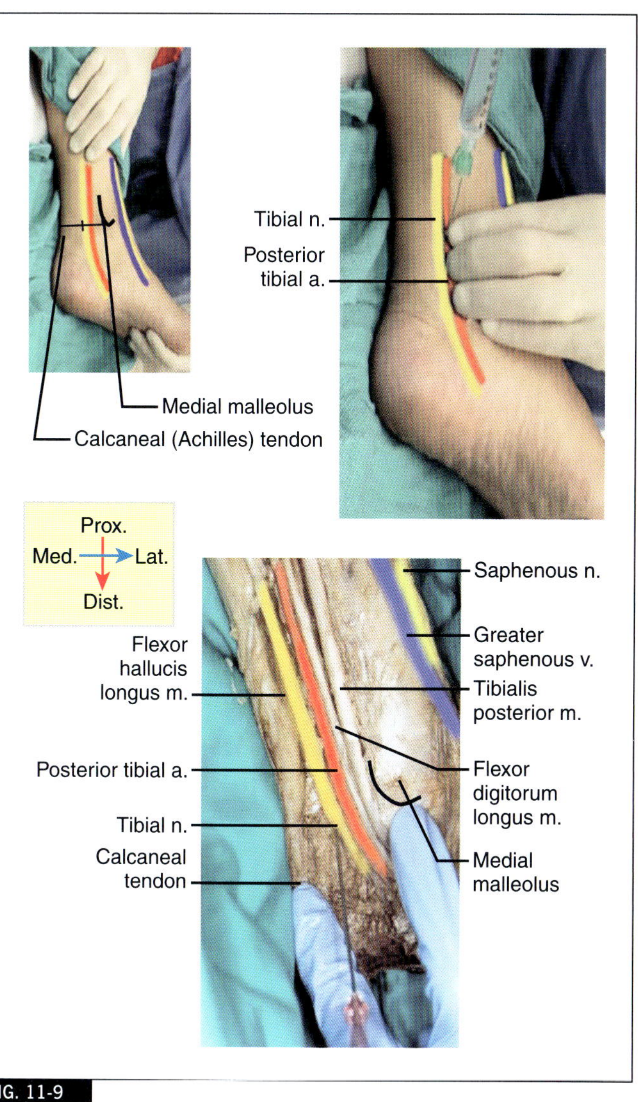

FIG. 11-9

Left ankle, tibial nerve block.

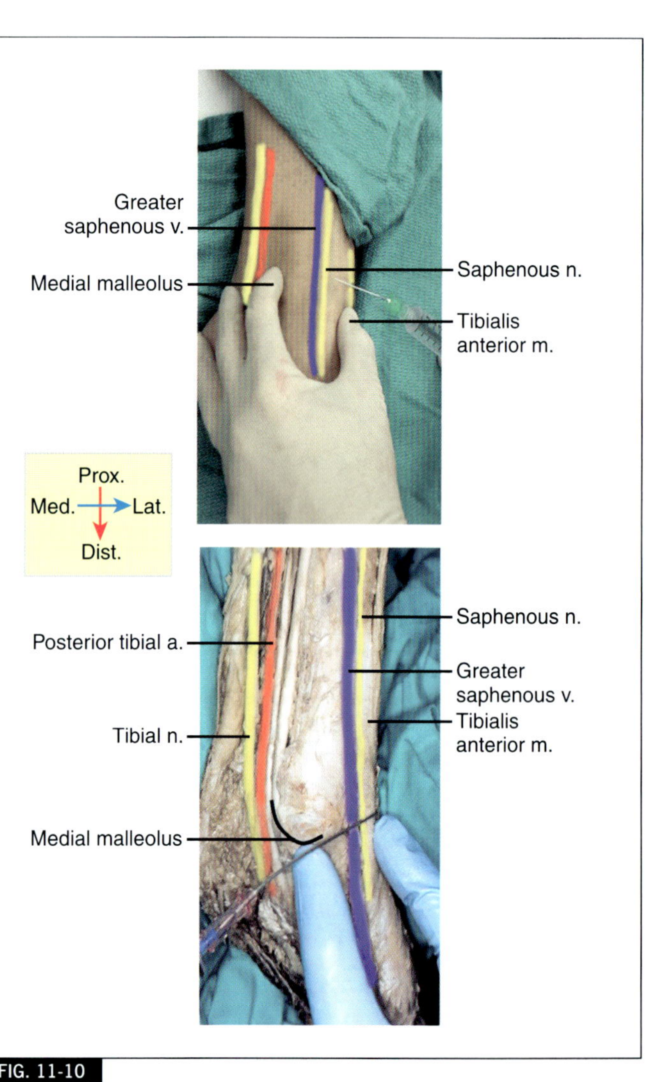

Left ankle, saphenous nerve block.

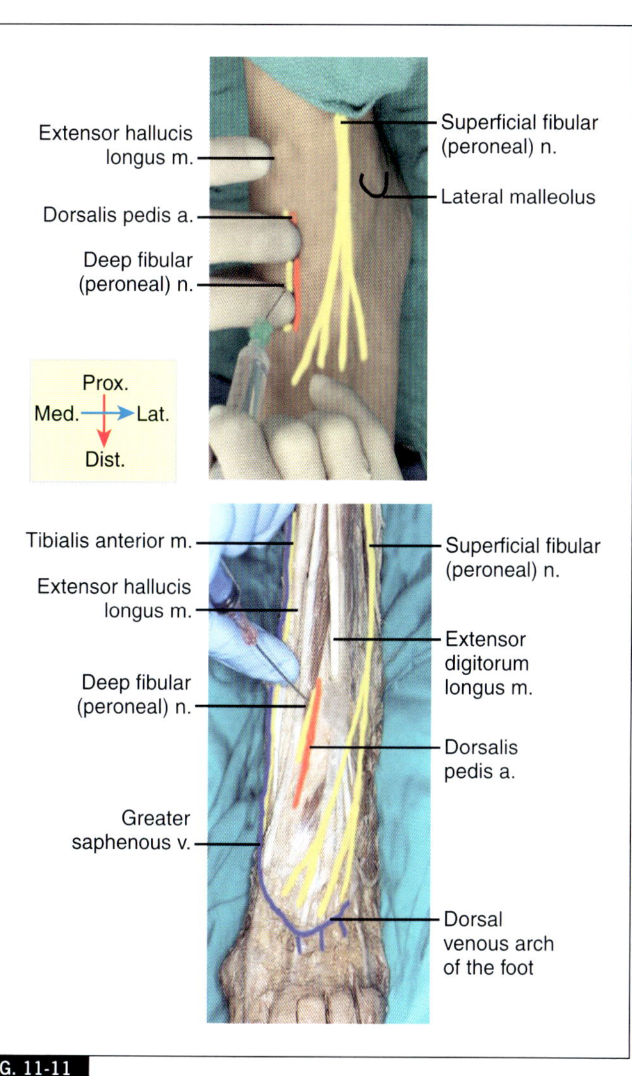

Left ankle, deep peroneal (fibular) nerve block.

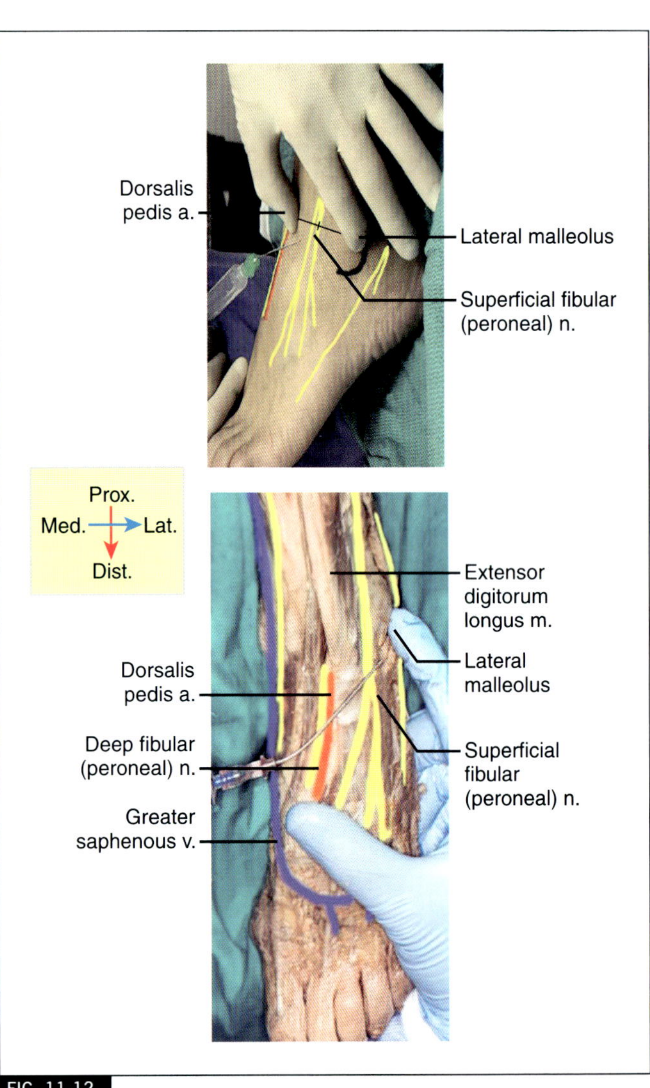

Left ankle, superficial peroneal (fibular) nerve block.

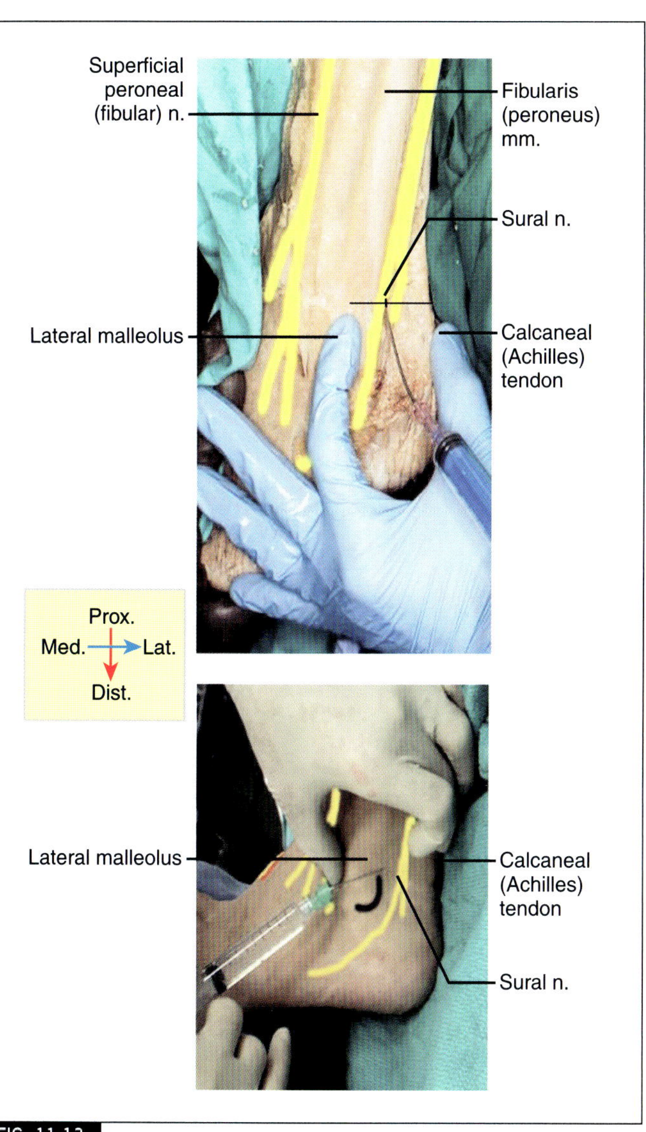

FIG. 11-13

Left ankle, sural nerve block.

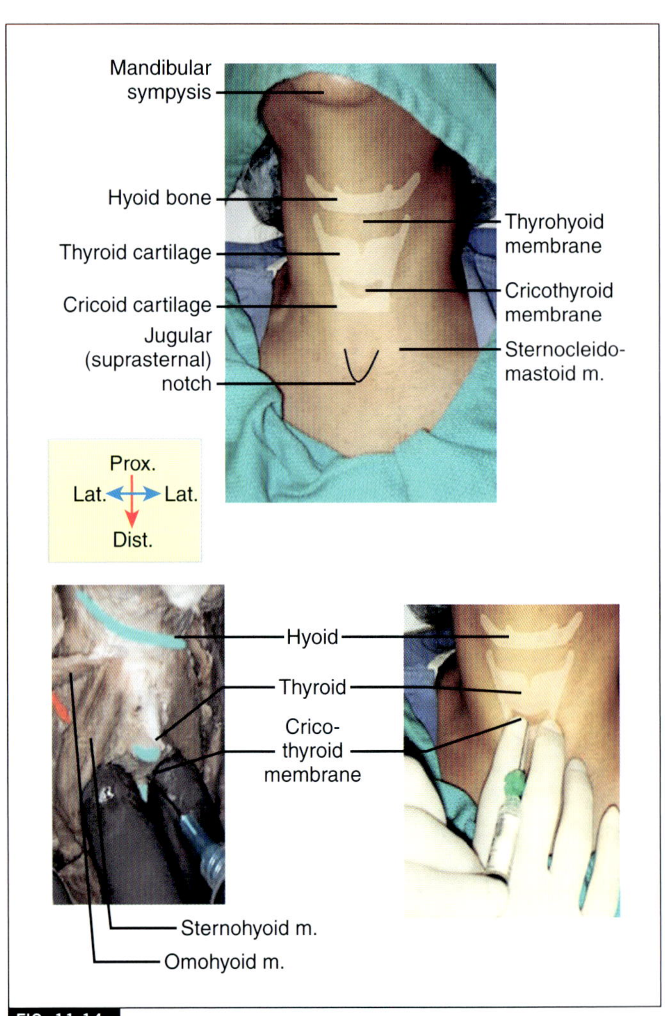

FIG. 11-14

Translaryngeal inferior laryngeal nerve block. ("Transtracheal")

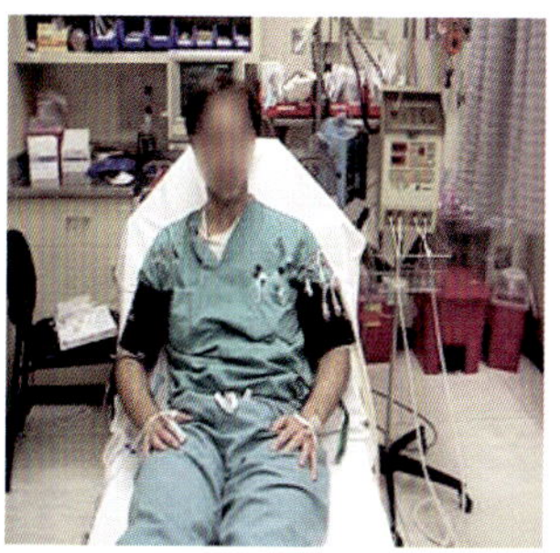

1. Oxygen and suction in readiness.
2. Patient monitors set up:
   - Blood pressure cuff
   - 3-lead ECG
   - Pulse oximeter
3. Emergency airway equipment available (see Chapter 5).
4. Intravenous line placed in the opposite side.
5. Heparin lock IV line placed in the operative side, as close to the injury site as possible.

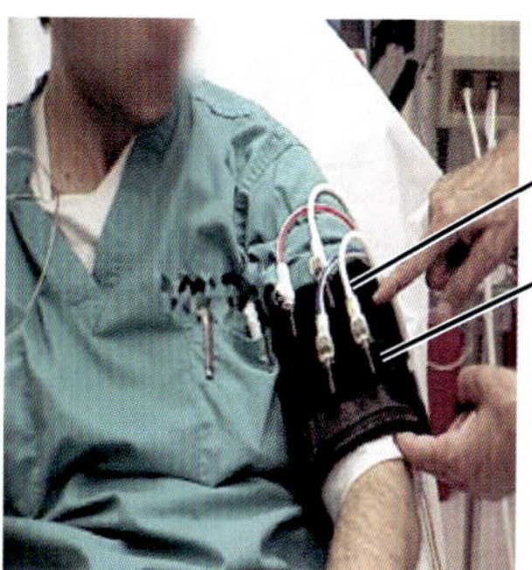

6. Double tourniquet snugly applied.
7. Check snugness with finger.

FIG. 11-15A

Bier block sequence.

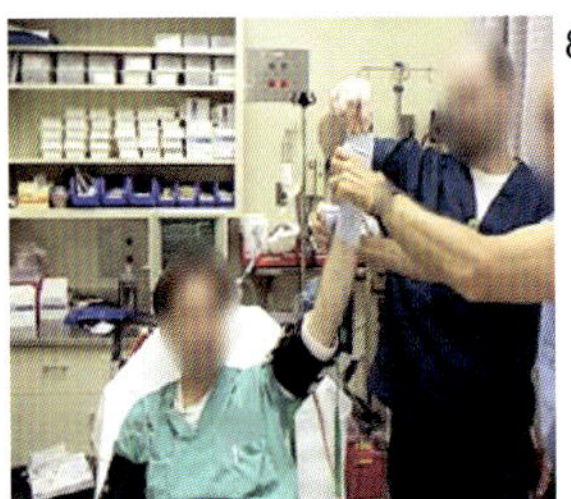

8. Exsanguinate the extremity from distal to proximal using an elastic bandage.

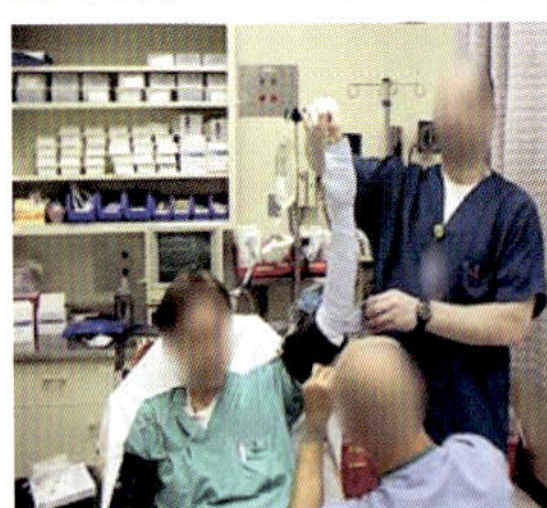

9. Inflate the **proximal** tourniquet to 100 mmHg above the systolic blood pressure.

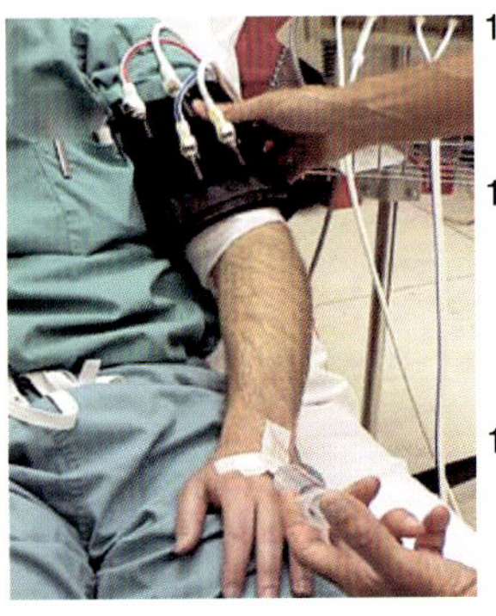

10. **Slowly** inject the local anesthetic. Expect a transient burning sensation and then venous engorgement.
11. If tourniquet pain begins prior to completion of the procedure, **inflate** the **distal** tourniquet (skin beneath should be numb) and then **deflate** the **proximal** tourniquet.
12. At the conclusion of the procedure, incrementally deflate the inflated tourniquets.

FIG. 11-15B

d. Bupivacaine 0.5% is chosen for a denser block: 0.5% = 5 mg/mL.
e. Femoral block requires 15 mL, so 15 mL × 5 mg/mL
   (0.5% bupivacaine) = 75 mg. This is well within maximum
   dose limits for infiltration and peripheral nerve block.
f. This amount could cause severe complications if accidentally injected
   intravascularly!
g. Typically, a 22-gauge, 1.5-inch needle is utilized for nerve blockade
   after sterile prep and drape and raising of a skin wheal with 1%
   lidocaine using a 25-gauge needle.

II. INDIVIDUAL NERVE BLOCKS

A. Neck, left side, superficial cervical plexus block (Fig. 11-1; see also Color Plate 11-1)

1. Indications: tracheostomy, superficial neck injury
2. Results:
a. Sensory block: left half of skin of neck
b. Motor block: none, if truly superficial

B. Left elbow

1. Median nerve block (Fig. 11-2; see also Color Plate 11-2)
a. Indications: hand analgesia and anesthesia
b. Results:
   (1) Sensory block: radial half of palmar skin, palmar skin of fingers 1–3 (4),
       dorsal skin of distal phalanges 1–3 (4)
   (2) Motor block: radial deviation of wrist; flexion, and opposition
       of thumb; weakened abduction of thumb; flexion of fingers
       1–3 (4)
2. Ulnar nerve block (Fig. 11-3; see also Color Plate 11-3)
a. Indications: hand and forearm analgesia and anesthesia
b. Results:
   (1) Sensory block: ulnar half of palmar skin; palmar and dorsal skin of
       fingers 4–5
   (2) Motor block: ulnar deviation of wrist; adduction of thumb; abduction
       and adduction of fingers, flexion and extension of fingers
c. Caveat: Make sure that anesthetic is administered proximal to the elbow,
   to avoid cubital tunnel syndrome.
3. Radial nerve block (Fig. 11-4; see also Color Plate 11-4)
a. Indications: hand and forearm analgesia and anesthesia
b. Results:
   (1) Sensory block: skin of thumb, radial half of dorsum of hand. Often
       lateral antebrachial cutaneous nerve is blocked as well, anesthetizing
       the lateral forearm.
   (2) Motor block: extension of wrist, supination of forearm may weaken,
       weakened abduction and extension of thumb, extension of fingers in
       the metacarpophalangeal joints.

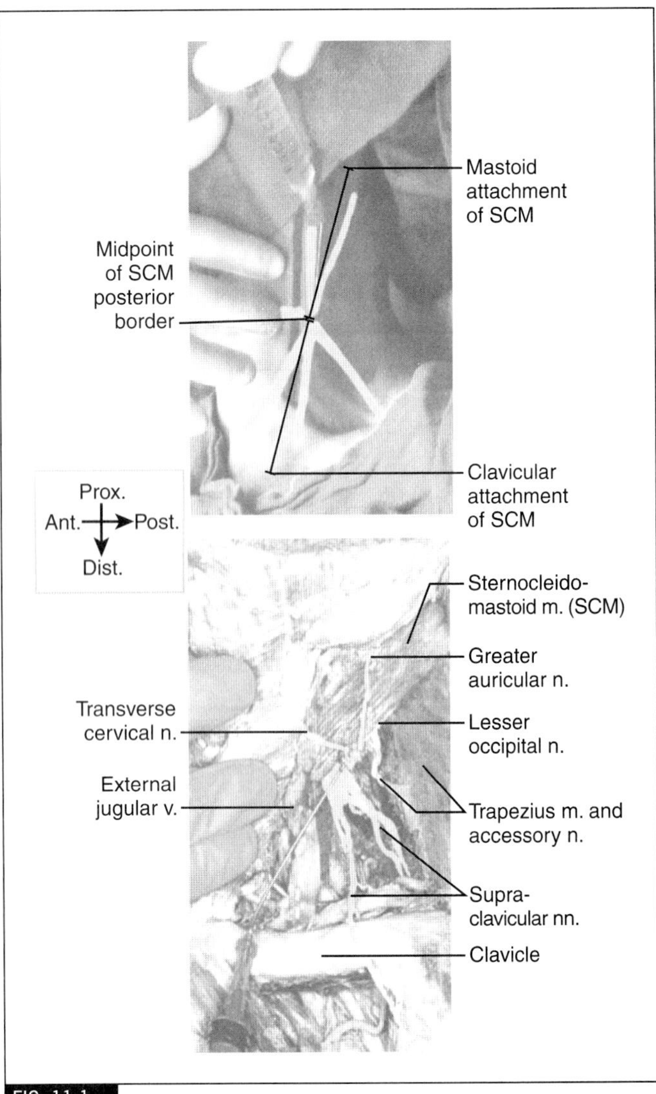

FIG. 11-1

Neck, left side, superficial cervical plexus block.

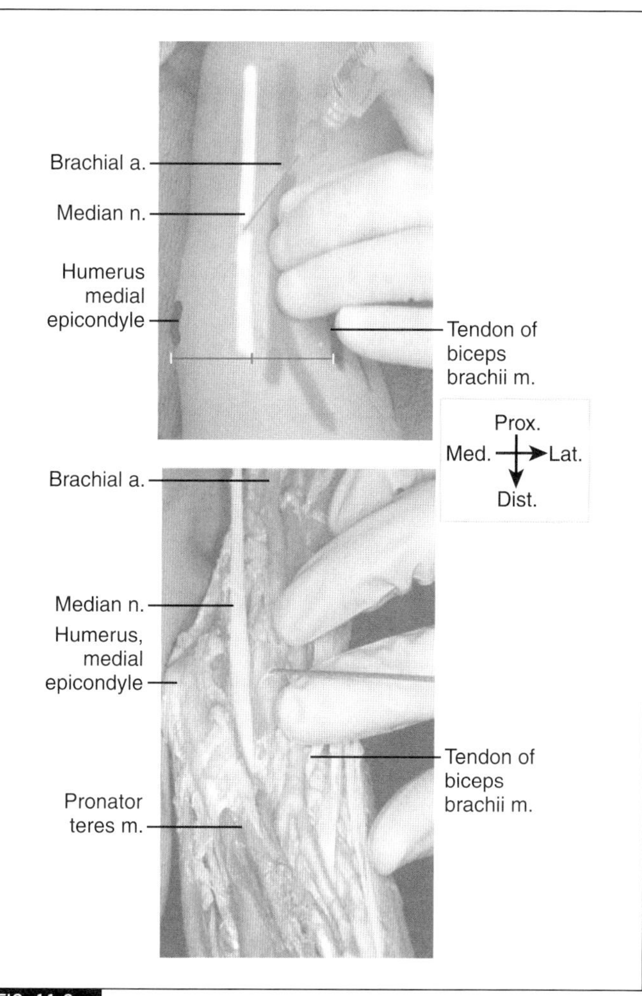

FIG. 11-2

Left elbow, median nerve block.

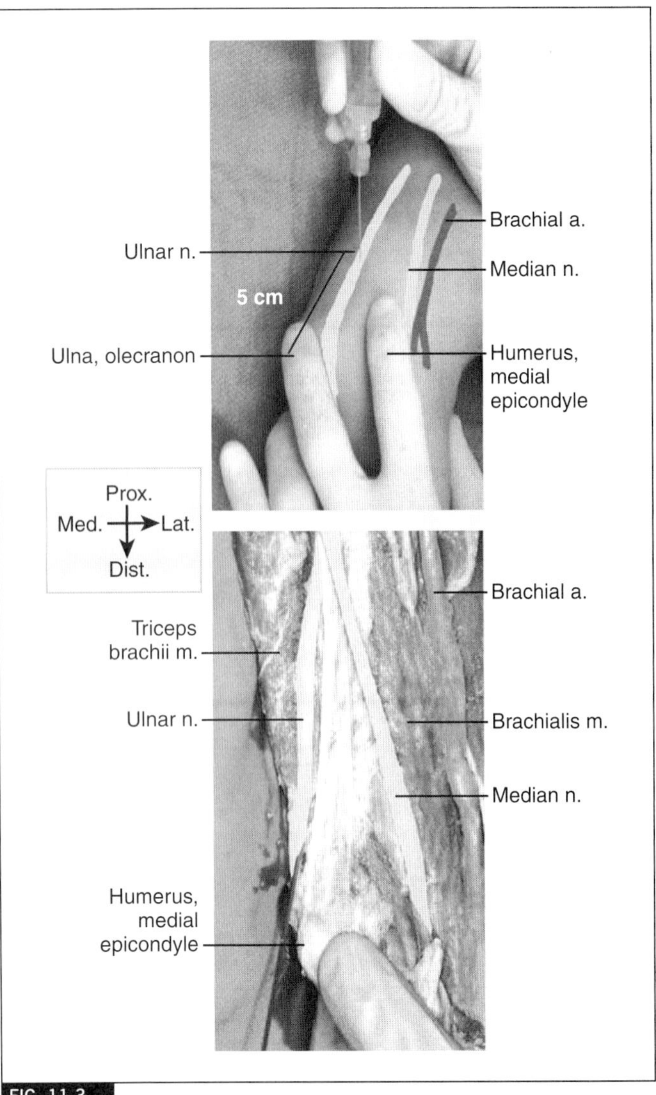

FIG. 11-3

Left elbow, ulnar nerve block.

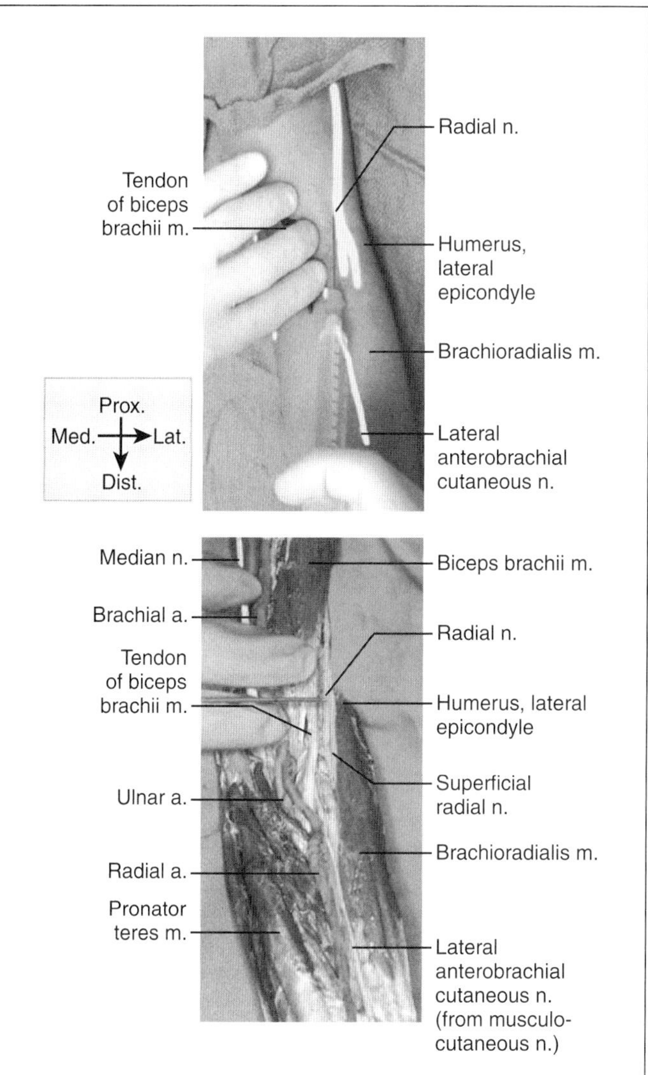

FIG. 11-4

Left elbow, radial nerve block.

c. Caveat: Make sure that anesthetic is administered proximal to the elbow to avoid radial tunnel syndrome.

C. Left wrist, forearm supinated
1. Median nerve block (Fig. 11-5; see also Color Plate 11-5)
a. Indications: first to third finger, thenar analgesia and anesthesia

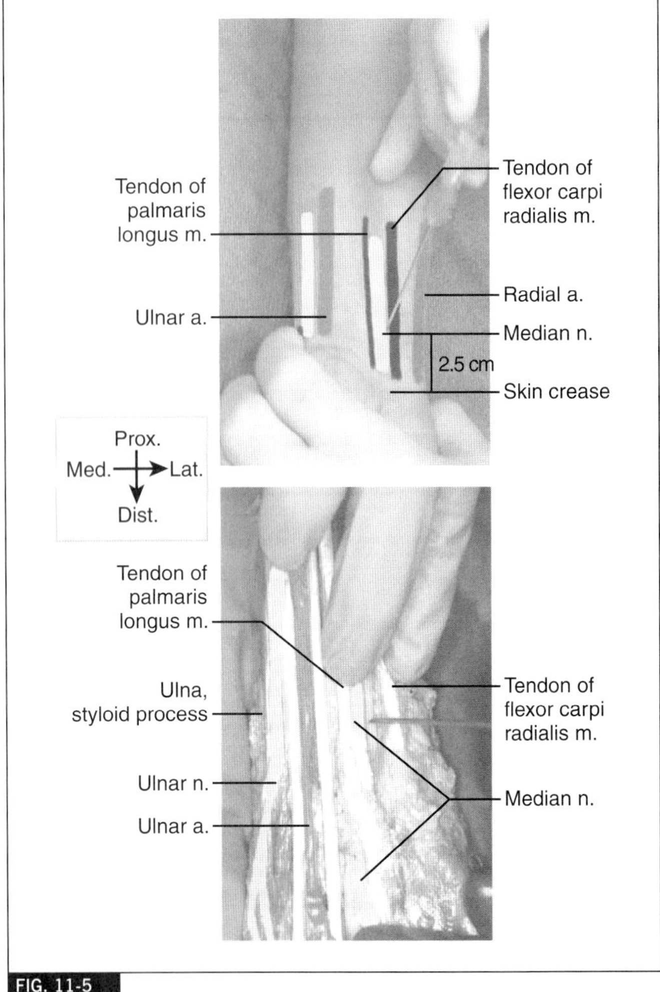

FIG. 11-5

Left wrist, forearm supinated, median nerve block.

b. Results:
   (1) Sensory block: palmar and dorsal skin of fingers 1–3 (4)
   (2) Motor block: opposition of thumb, weakened abduction of thumb
c. Caveat: Make sure that anesthetic is administered proximal to the wrist to avoid carpal tunnel syndrome.
2. Ulnar nerve block (Fig. 11-6; see also Color Plate 11-6)
a. Indications: fourth to fifth finger, hypothenar analgesia and anesthesia
b. Results:
   (1) Sensory block: ulnar half of palmar skin, palmar skin of fingers
      4–5
   (2) Motor block: abduction and adduction of fingers
c. Caveat: Make sure that anesthetic is administered proximal to the wrist to avoid tunnel syndrome at Guyon's canal.

D. Left hand, digital nerve block of the middle finger
1. The upper image in Figure 11-7 (see also Color Plate 11-7) shows the forearm pronated, dorsal view; the lower image shows the forearm supinated, palmar (volar) view.
2. Indications: finger anesthesia and analgesia
3. Results:
a. Sensory block: skin of middle finger. Two injections applied approaching finger from dorsal: one on radial and one on ulnar aspect, at the metacarpophalangeal web space
b. Motor block: NONE
4. Caveat: NEVER add epinephrine to local anesthetic when performing a finger block.

E. Left femoral triangle, femoral nerve block (Fig. 11-8; see also Color Plate 11-8)
1. Indications: Femur anesthesia (higher volume may block entire lumbar plexus and anesthetize the hip), moderate knee analgesia
2. Results:
a. Sensory block: anterior aspect of thigh, anteromedial aspect of leg. May cause anesthesia of the medial and lateral thigh and part of the buttocks.
b. Motor block: extension and lateral rotation of the knee joint. May prevent adduction and abduction of the hip joint.
3. Caveat: Aspirate carefully to avoid injury to the femoral artery.

F. Left ankle
1. Tibial nerve block (Fig. 11-9; see also Color Plate 11-9)
a. Indications: medial foot analgesia and anesthesia
b. Results:
   (1) Sensory block: sole of foot except lateral aspect, and plantar aspect of toes
   (2) Motor block: abduction of big toe, weakened flexion of toes

11   COMMON NERVE BLOCKS

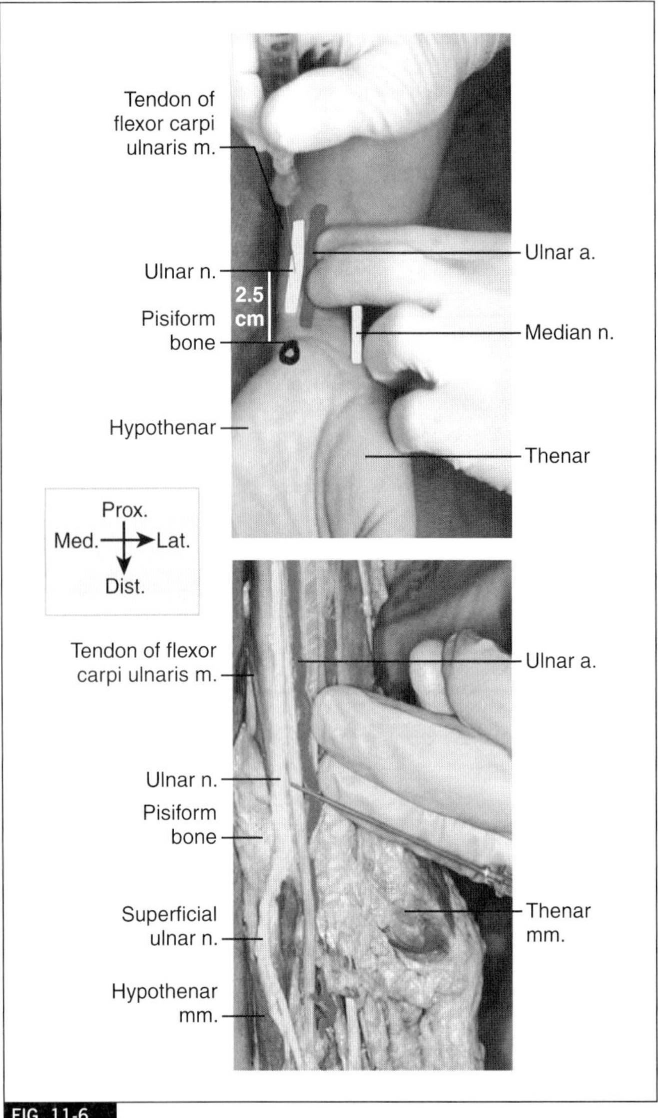

FIG. 11-6

Left wrist, forearm supinated, ulnar nerve block.

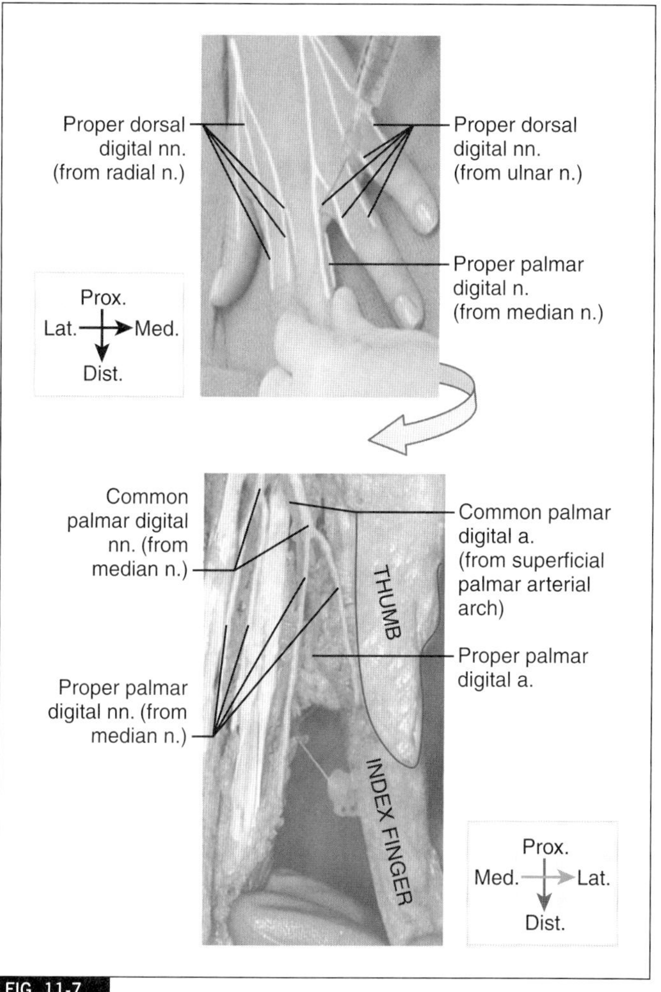

FIG. 11-7

Left hand, digital nerve block of middle finger. *Upper image*, Forearm pronated, dorsal view. *Lower image*, Forearm supinated, palmar (volar) view.

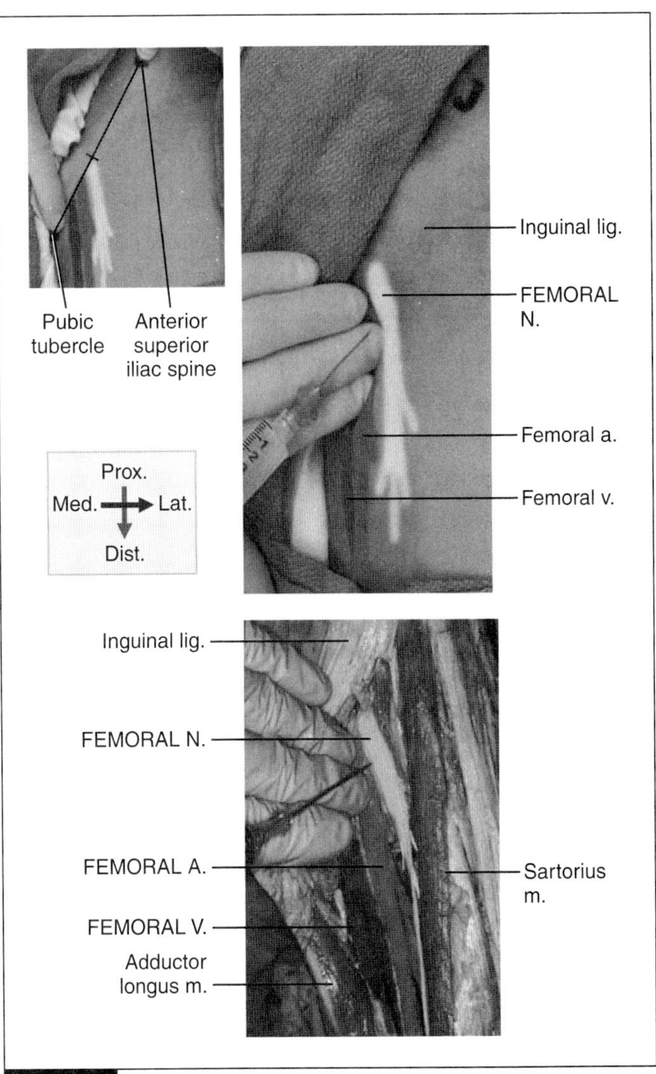

FIG. 11-8

Left femoral triangle, femoral nerve block.

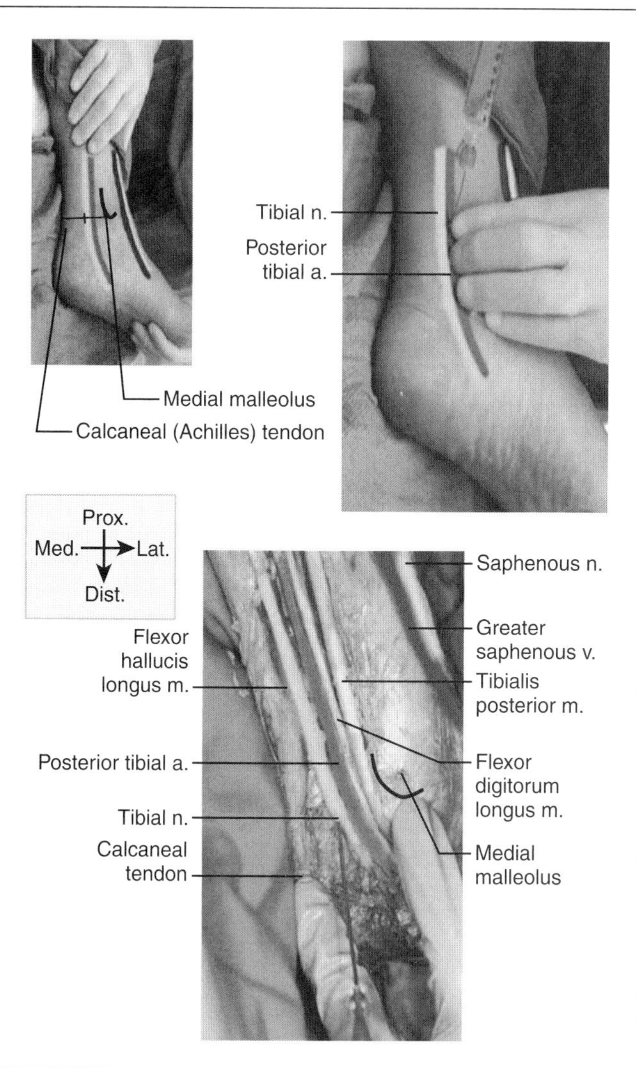

FIG. 11-9

Left ankle, tibial nerve block.

2. Saphenous nerve block (Fig. 11-10; see also Color Plate 11-10)
a. Indications: field block, medial ankle and big toe anesthesia
b. Results:
    (1) Sensory block: medial ankle
    (2) Motor block: NONE

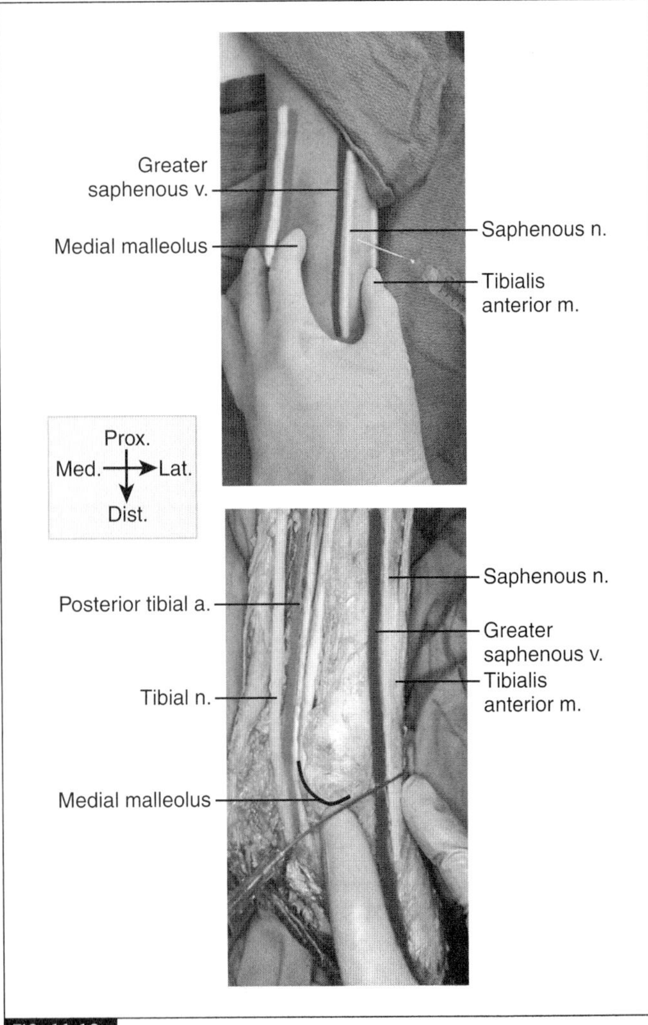

FIG. 11-10

Left ankle, saphenous nerve block.

3. Deep peroneal (fibular) nerve block (Fig. 11-11; see also Color Plate 11-11)
a. Indications: first web space anesthesia
b. Results:
   (1) Sensory block: web space between big toe and toe 2
   (2) Motor block: weakened extension of toes

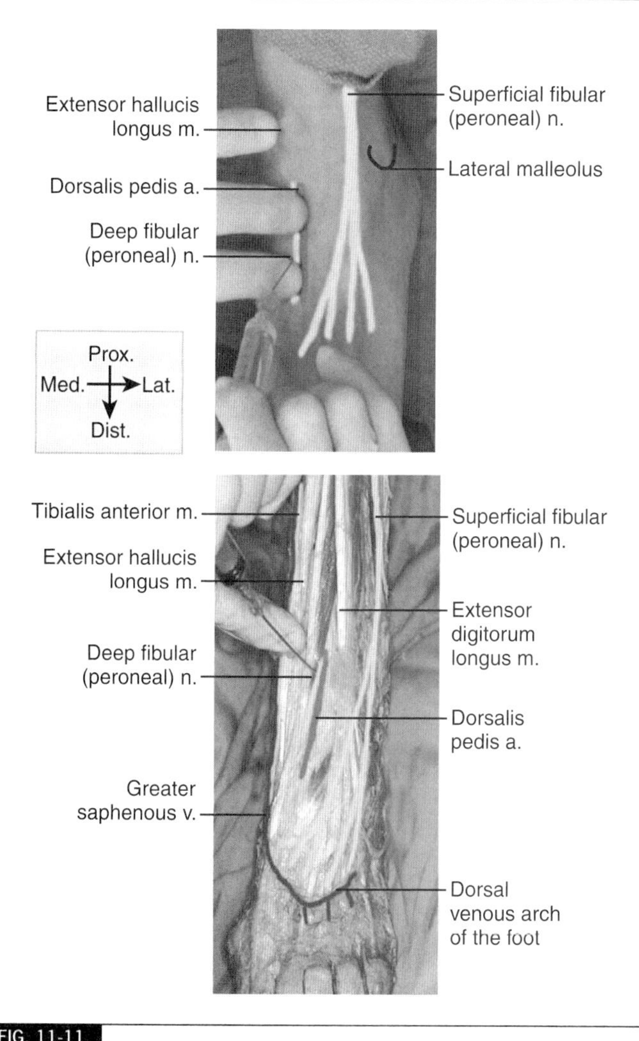

FIG. 11-11

Left ankle, deep peroneal (fibular) nerve block.

4. Superficial peroneal (fibular) nerve block (Fig. 11-12; see also Color Plate 11-12)
a. Indications: field block, dorsal foot anesthesia
b. Results:
   (1) Sensory block: dorsum of foot and toes
   (2) Motor block: NONE
5. Sural nerve block (Fig. 11-13; see also Color Plate 11-13)
a. Indications: field block, lateral foot anesthesia
b. Results:
   (1) Sensory block: lateral ankle, lateral aspect of dorsum and sole of foot
   (2) Motor block: NONE

G. Translaryngeal ("Transtracheal") inferior laryngeal nerve block
   (Fig. 11-14; see also Color Plate 11–14)
1. Indications: intubation in awake patient
2. Results:
a. Sensory block: below vocal cords to carina of trachea
b. Motor block: NONE

H. Bier block sequence and intravenous regional anesthesia
1. This represents a very useful technique for anesthetizing the more distal aspects of an extremity for procedures such as dislocation reduction, fracture manipulation, and complex laceration repair.
2. The technique involves injecting a local anesthetic in a distal extremity vein AFTER isolating the vasculature with a PROXIMAL tourniquet. By slowly injecting the local anesthetic, most of the injected dose remains confined to the extremity and flows into the nerves through vascular channels that penetrate the epineurium.
3. Extremity anesthesia is established from distal to proximal.
4. The block would theoretically last indefinitely because the local anesthetic cannot reach the liver to be metabolized.
5. *Practically, the block is limited by tourniquet pain, which generally becomes intolerable after 30 minutes.*
6. Local anesthetic choice is limited to those agents in concentrations that would not cause catastrophic cardiovascular collapse in the event of tourniquet leak or failure (bupivacaine). The most commonly used agent is **lidocaine 0.5%.**
7. Local anesthetic-induced systemic symptoms are still possible when the tourniquet is deflated, and most practitioners feel that minimum tourniquet time should be 15 minutes to allow more of the agent to fix in the tissues so that a systemic bolus is not released. An added safety measure at the conclusion of the procedure is intermittently deflating and inflating the tourniquet for several 10 second cycles while monitoring for systemic symptoms.
8. Typical volumes are 30 to 40 mL for the arm and 50 to 70 mL for the leg. The leg is technically much more difficult due to cuff and tourniquet fit issues and volume and concentration of local anesthetic required.

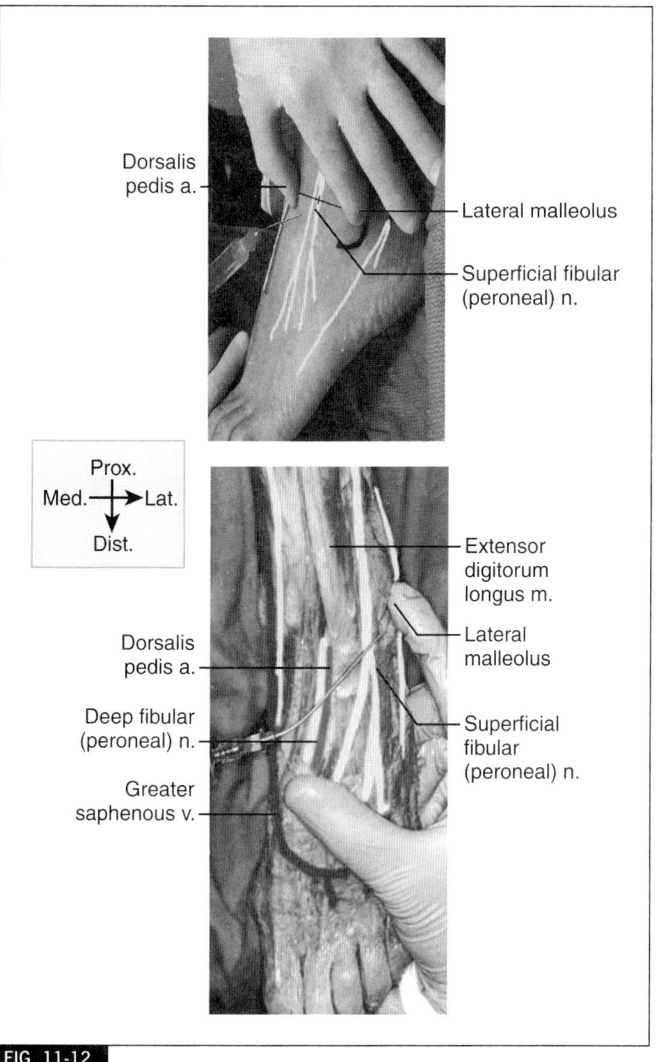

FIG. 11-12

Left ankle, superficial peroneal (fibular) nerve block.

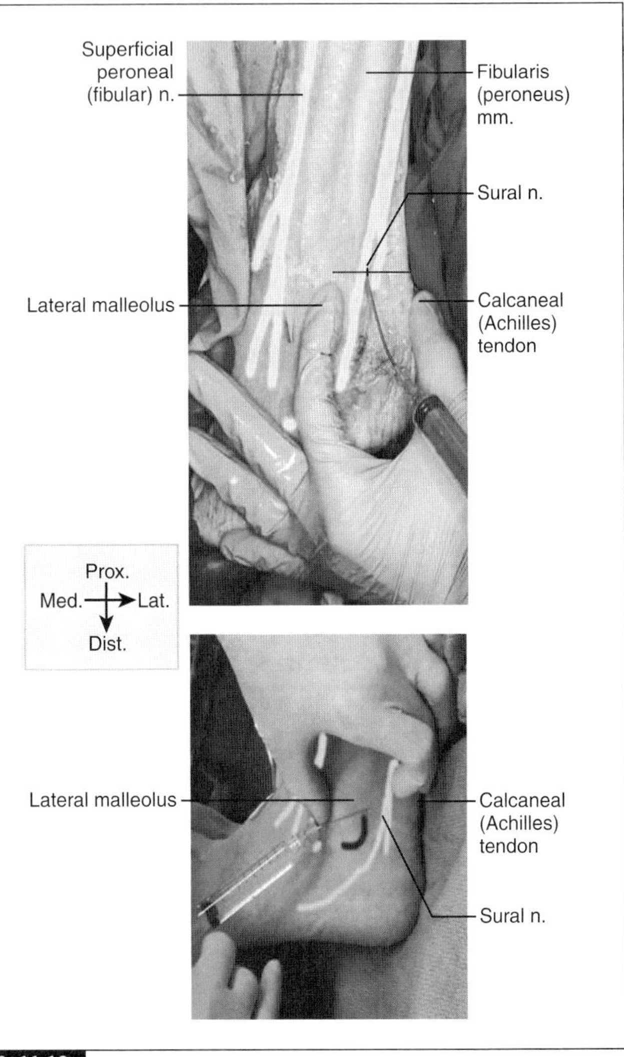

FIG. 11-13

Left ankle, sural nerve block.

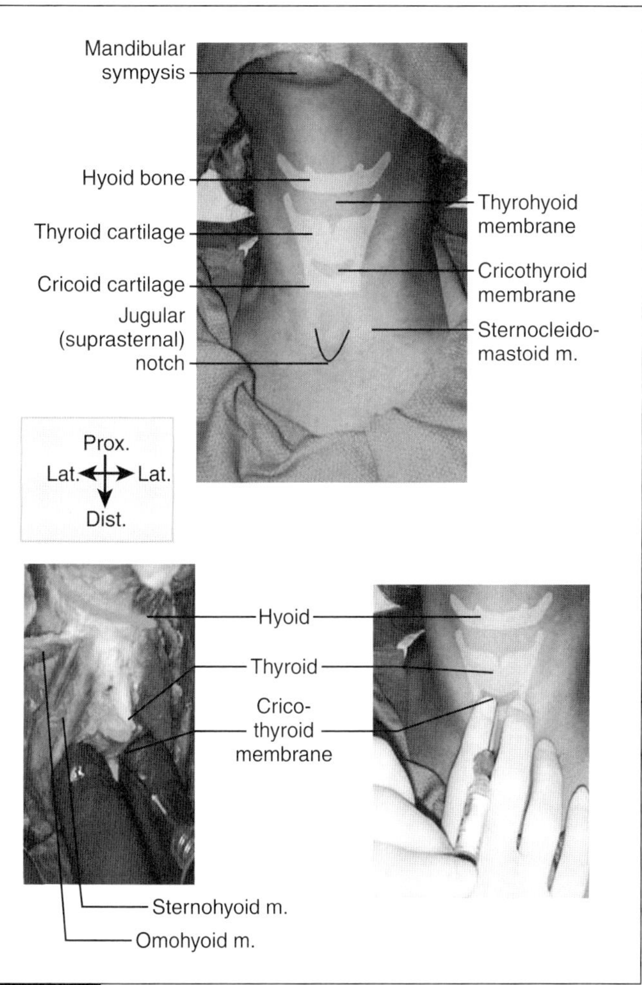

FIG. 11-14

Translaryngeal inferior laryngeal nerve block. ("Transtracheal")

9. Technique
a. Full monitors (blood pressure cuff, electrocardiogram, pulse oximeter)
   Available oxygen and suction
b. IV line placed in the opposite side (Fig. 11-15A; see also Color Plate
   11-15A)
c. Heparin lock IV in the operative side, as close to the injury site as
   possible

d. Double tourniquet snugly applied
e. Exsanguinate the extremity from distal to proximal using an elastic bandage (see Fig. 11-15B; see also Color Plate 11-15B).
f. Inflate the PROXIMAL tourniquet to 100 mm Hg above the systolic blood pressure.
g. SLOWLY inject the local anesthetic. Expect a transient burning sensation and then venous engorgement.
h. If tourniquet pain begins before completion of the procedure, INFLATE the DISTAL tourniquet (skin beneath should be numb) and then DEFLATE the PROXIMAL tourniquet.
i. Incrementally deflate the inflated tourniquet at the conclusion of the procedure.

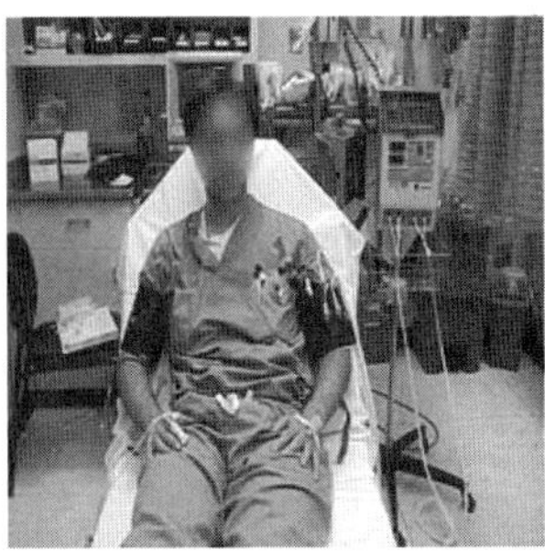

1. Oxygen and suction in readiness.
2. Patient monitors set up:
   - Blood pressure cuff
   - 3-lead ECG
   - Pulse oximeter
3. Emergency airway equipment available (see Chapter 5).
4. Intravenous line placed in the opposite side
5. Heparin lock IV line placed in the operative side, as close to the injury site as possible

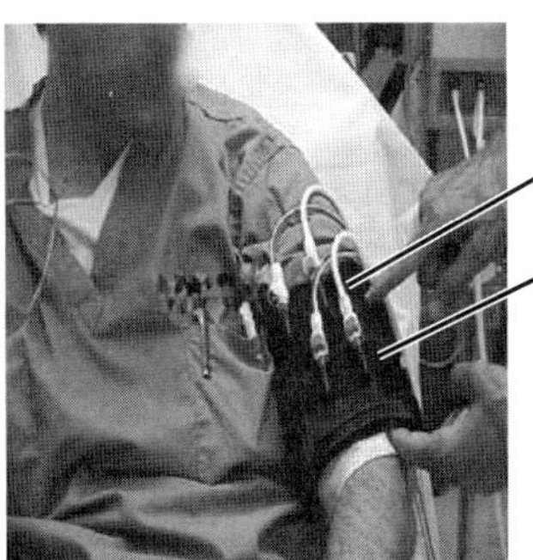

6. Double tourniquet snugly applied
7. Check snugness with finger.

A

FIG. 11-15A

Bier block sequence. *(Continued)*

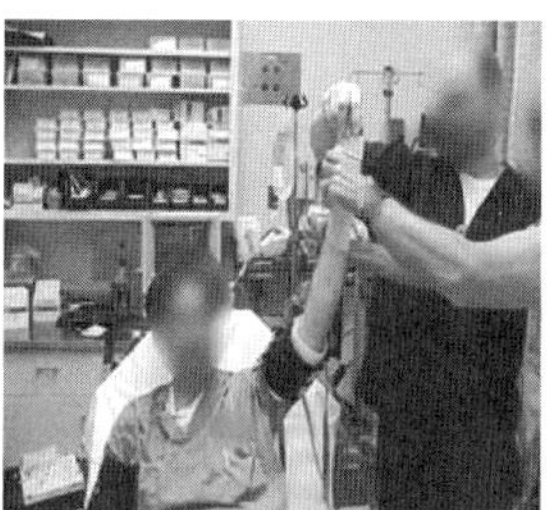

8. Exsanguinate the extremity from distal to proximal using an elastic bandage.

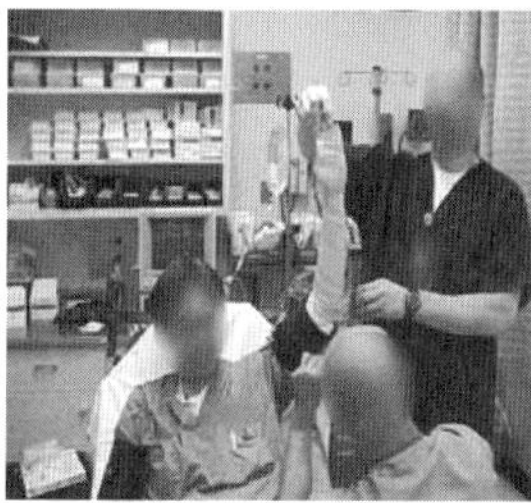

9. Inflate the **proximal** tourniquet to 100 mmHg above the systolic blood pressure.

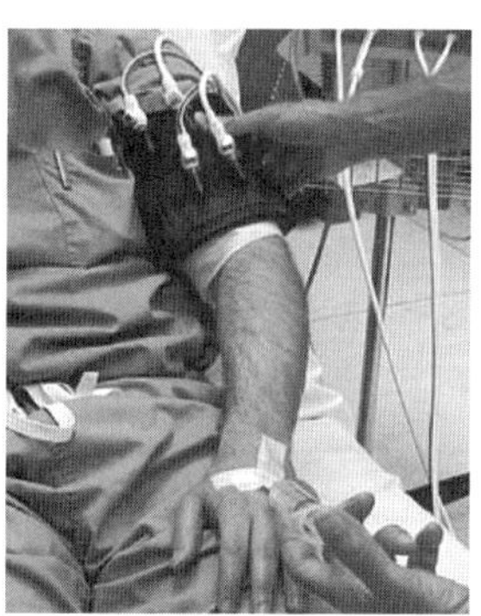

10. **Slowly** inject the local anesthetic. Expect a transient burning sensation and then venous engorgement.
11. If tourniquet pain begins prior to completion of the procedure, **inflate** the **distal** tourniquet (skin beneath should be numb) and then **deflate** the **proximal** tourniquet.
12. At the conclusion of the procedure, incrementally deflate the inflated tourniquets.

B

FIG. 11-15B

10. Drug calculation
  a. Lidocaine: 70 kg patient
      (1) Upper extremity volume = 40 mL
      (2) Safe dose for lidocaine for Bier block = 2 to 3 mg/kg

Note: *This is lower than for infiltration and nerve block anesthesia!*

(3) 70 kg patient = 3 mg/kg × 70 kg = 210 mg

(4) 210 mg/40 mL = approx. × 5 mg/mL = 0.5%

b. Mixture: 20 mL 1% lidocaine + 20 mL 0.9% NaCl *OR* 10 mL 2% lidocaine + 30 mL 0.9% NaCl

c. Caveats:

(1) Start with volume required and maximum safe dose and then calculate mixture.

(2) Always use preservative-free mixtures to avoid possible methylparaben allergy.

(3) Be careful with drug calculations!

(4) Ensure snug, functioning tourniquet.

(5) Tourniquet should remain inflated for at least 15 minutes.

(6) Most likely local anesthetic: Reactions on deflation are central nervous system related—dysarthria, lightheadedness, tinnitus, and so forth. Be ready to treat.

(7) Inject solution slowly; rapid injection can overpower the tourniquet through deep muscular venous channels.

(8) Avoid bupivacaine; NO epinephrine!

Analgesia and Sedation in Special Populations

W. James Phillips

12

I. ELDERLY PATIENTS

A. Physiologic changes associated with aging

1. Include a gradual decline in organ system function, typically manifested as *loss of functional reserve.*
2. System specific changes include:
a. Cardiovascular: increased myocardial stiffness, decreased response to catecholamines with a 1% drop in cardiac index/year
b. Respiratory: gradual loss of elasticity, gradual increased ventilation-perfusion mismatch, age-related restrictive mechanics
c. Renal: 1% decline in glomerular density/year, gradual decline in renal blood flow
d. Hepatic: gradual decline in hepatic blood flow, tissue mass, and enzyme function
e. Nervous system: gradual loss of neuronal density, decreased conduction in peripheral nerves, blunted baroreceptor responses to fluid volume changes, increased basal sympathetic nervous system activity, exaggerated response to central nervous system (CNS) depressants
f. Vascular system: decreased blood volume, decreased protein binding

B. Drug choices in elderly patients

1. Acetaminophen: probably the drug of choice for initial management of mild pain. Avoid doses > 3 to 4 g/day.
2. Nonsteroidal anti-inflammatory drugs (NSAIDs): All NSAIDS (nonselective and cyclooxygenase-2 [COX-2]) inhibitors carry the risk of renal dysfunction, hypertension, fluid retention, platelet inhibition, and gastrointestinal (GI) bleeding.
3. COX-2 inhibitors: celecoxib (Celebrex) and valdecoxib (Bextra)
a. May offer a decreased risk for GI bleeding and platelet dysfunction, but at the expense of potentially **increasing cardiovascular risk**. This is likely due to a relative inhibition of prostacyclin I (vasodilator), leaving thromboxane A_2 (vasoconstrictor, platelet aggregator) undisturbed.
b. One should think twice about using these agents in elderly patients with a history of hypertension, diabetes mellitus, or peptic ulcer disease.

Note: *There is also no analgesic superiority of COX-2 inhibitors over the nonselective NSAIDs.*

c. Parecoxib is the water-soluble prodrug of valdecoxib and is the only available (Europe) parenteral COX-2 inhibitor.

4. Opiates
a. Elderly patients may exhibit an exaggerated and prolonged response to oral and parenteral opiates. This is likely due to:
   (1) Decreases in receptor density
   (2) Decreases in protein binding
   (3) Decreased hepatic and renal blood flow
b. Consider a 20% decrease in starting opiate doses for each decade after age 60 years.
c. One may also consider increasing the dosing interval by 20% to 30%.
d. Beware exaggerated respiratory depression, constipation, and additive sedation with other CNS depressants.
e. Advantages of carefully titrated dose of opiates in elderly patients are a general lack of organ toxicity as compared with the NSAIDs.
5. Co-analgesics: The most commonly employed agents are the tricyclic antidepressants and the anticonvulsants for neuropathic pain syndromes such as peripheral neuropathy and postherpetic neuralgia.
a. Tricyclic antidepressants: Although useful, the anticholinergic effects may exacerbate arrhythmia tendencies, constipation, prostatism, glaucoma, and orthostasis. Desipramine may carry the lowest anticholinergic risk of these agents. Nortriptyline (Pamelor) is the active metabolite of amitriptyline and is another useful agent at low starting doses of 10 to 25 mg PO at bedtime.
b. The selective serotonin reuptake blockers have little documented efficacy for neuropathic pain.
c. Of the anticonvulsants, gabapentin (Neurontin) and pregabalin (Lyrica) may be the best tolerated agents. Gabapentin is also devoid of organ toxicity, but the **dosage must be drastically reduced in cases of renal insufficiency.**
d. A conservative gabapentin regimen in elderly patients would be 100 to 300 mg PO twice daily, then three times daily with a dose escalation of 300 mg every 3–5 days to a maximum of 3000 mg/day.
6. Procedural sedation choices
a. Although all parenteral sedatives may be carefully employed in elderly patients, etomidate is likely the drug of choice because of its relative hemodynamic stability. Precipitous hypotension is common with propofol and the barbiturates. Prolonged effects are not unusual.
b. Liberal use of other analgesic techniques such as IV regional anesthesia or peripheral nerve blockage should be employed when applicable.

II. PATIENTS WITH RENAL INSUFFICIENCY OR FAILURE

A. Pharmacokinetic changes seen with decreased real function include:
1. Decreased GI absorption of drugs
2. Increased initial volume of distribution (Vd) due to edema
3. Decreased Vd due to decreased muscle mass
4. Decreased drug protein binding due to decreased albumin and albumin affinity

5. Decreased renal drug secretion (tubular)
6. Decreased renal drug excretion (glomerular)
7. Decreased first-pass *hepatic* metabolism
8. Decreased drug reduction or hydrolysis

B. Start by:
This can be confusing ...
1. Assessing the state of hydration
2. Ideal body weight (IBW)
a. Males—50 kg + 2.3 kg/inch over 5 feet
b. Females—45.5 kg + 2.3 kg/inch over 5 feet
3. Calculate creatinine clearance (CRCL): Cockroft and Gault equation
a. CRCL = (140 − age) × IBW (kg)/72 × serum creatinine
   (× 0.85 for women)
4. Get a sense of fitness and muscle mass; that is, a normal creatinine
   may be *abnormal* in the cachectic debilitated patient.
5. Remember that *loading doses* are the same (or *increased* if edema is
   present) in cases of renal insufficiency (unless the patient is
   cachectic)
6. Dosing intervals will be changed.
7. Avoid drugs with any significant renal excretion (if possible)
8. Understand that dialysis is less able to remove drugs with a high Vd
   (extensively tissue bound), high protein binding (>80%), and high
   molecular weight (>1500 to 2000 dalton). *Vd is the most important
   of these factors.*
9. In the presence of renal insufficiency, one may elect to lower the
   maintenance dose, increase the dosing interval, or combine the two.
10. Dosing *may* remain normal as long as the CRCL remains >50 mL/min.

C. Choosing an analgesic
1. Oral: Oxycodone (e.g., Percocet, Tylox) is a reasonable choice. Codeine
   is an acceptable alternative. Consider ½ typical doses when CRCL < 50
   mL/min.
2. Parenteral and patient-controlled analgesia use: Hydromorphone and
   Fentanyl are good choices. Although minimal renal excretion occurs,
   consider ½ typical doses when CRCL < 50 mL/min.
3. Avoid meperidine, morphine, propoxyphene (active metabolites renally
   excreted).
4. Remember: Renal patients may be more prone to global sedative effect
   of opiates.
5. Other drug caveats:
a. Gabapentin dose must be markedly reduced with renal insufficiency.
b. Hydroxyzine (Vistaril) dose must be reduced.

D. Choosing a procedural sedative
1. Propofol, the barbiturates, ketamine, and etomidate are all acceptable
   choices. Despite a lack of renal excretion, conservative dosing must be

used because of increased cardiovascular and CNS sensitivity to these agents.
2. The dose of midazolam requires significant decreases with lower creatinine clearances. Etomidate and ketamine may be particularly useful given the decreased tendency for *hypotension*.
3. Remember also that time to peak drug effect may be altered because of changes in Vd. Patience and careful titration are critical.

III. PATIENTS WITH HEPATIC INSUFFICIENCY

A. Overview

1. Because the liver has such substantial reserve, hepatic cellular loss will be far advanced before being clinically apparent. Waxing and waning damage is best followed by bilirubin and enzyme testing. There is no good test for assessing excretion and detoxification function and the synthetic markers of serum albumin and the prothrombin time are used as surrogate tests. As liver function further declines, the blood urea nitrogen (BUN) level may drop because of an inability of the liver to convert ammonia to urea. Further loss of hepatic function may result in hypoglycemic episodes as a result of an inability to mobilize glucose from glycogen or perform gluconeogenesis.
2. Significant loss of hepatic architecture causes portal venous hypertension, fluid retention, hyponatremia, and an elevation of total body water. This creates a larger Vd for many agents, thus compounding the delay in transport to the liver for metabolism.
3. When choosing a sedative or analgesic, it is essential to remember that essentially all opiate analgesics and procedural sedation agents undergo all or part of their metabolism in the liver.
4. NSAIDs are likewise problematic because of the increased incidence of adverse effects in cases of decreased circulatory plasma volume (e.g., liver disease, congestive heart failure).
5. The following phenomena may be experienced when administering sedatives and analgesics to the patient with impaired liver function:
a. Larger initial dose required
b. Delayed onset
c. More profound cardiovascular depression due to diminished intravascular volume
d. Exaggerated sedative effects of both analgesics and procedural sedatives
e. Prolonged recovery times from both analgesics and/or sedative agents

B. An approach to drug dosing may be:

1. Calculate IBW
a. Males—50 kg + 2.3 kg/inch over 5 feet
b. Females—45.5 kg + 2.3 kg/inch over 5 feet
2. Assess degree of hydration and total body water, taking into account serum sodium.

3. *Roughly* estimate hepatic synthetic function by serum albumin.
4. Decrease calculated IBW doses by the percentage decreases in serum albumin from normal, that is, serum albumin 50% normal = starting drug dose decreased 50%.
5. For analgesics, consider also increasing the *dose interval* to allow for delayed metabolism.
6. Consider avoidance of long-acting agents such as MS Contin, methadone, and OxyContin.

IV. PATIENTS WITH TENUOUS CARDIAC STATUS

A. Some examples of this situation include patients requiring cardioversion, congestive heart failure requiring sedation for intubation, hip relocation in the elderly patient with marginal cardiac reserve, and procedural sedation in the patient with uncontrolled hypertension or angina.

B. Approach
1. Optimize oxygenation and hydration through fluid bolus therapy versus diuretic, preoxygenation, and so forth.
2. Consider arterial line placement for beat-to-beat blood pressure (BP) control.
3. Consider BP control need for cardioprotective agents such as β blockers. Titrate to optimal target heart rate and BP.
4. Consider a regional analgesia technique such as:
a. Airway anesthesia for awake intubation
b. Femoral nerve block for femur fracture management
c. Bier block for wrist reduction
5. If parenteral sedation is required, consider:
a. Fentanyl in doses of 25 to 50 μg at a time until modest sedation is attained; *OR*
b. Etomidate in 2- to 4-mg increments IV until adequate sedation is obtained.
c. Both of these agents offer excellent hemodynamic stability and can be titrated to give **sedation without apnea.**

V. PATIENTS WITH INCREASED INTRACRANIAL PRESSURE

A. Examples of this situation include sedation for intubation and fracture manipulation in the head injury patient.

B. Intubation and mechanical ventilation are often inevitable in patients with elevated intracranial pressure (ICP).

C. Because cerebral perfusion pressure (CPP) = mean arterial pressure (MAP) − ICP (estimated by central venous pressure [CVP]), the goal is to administer sedative agents that lower ICP without much drop in BP so that cerebral perfusion pressure is maintained.

D. Agents that lower ICP do so by lowering cerebral metabolic rate and thereby causing a reflex cerebral vasoconstriction.
1. These "cerebral vasoconstrictors" may include:
a. Barbiturates
b. Etomidate
c. Propofol
d. Opiates
e. Benzodiazepines
2. Barbiturates are the gold standard for cerebral protection but often cause unacceptable drops in BP. Remember that a single episode of hypotension has been associated with worsened outcomes in the presence of elevated ICP!
3. Propofol is similar in this regard.
4. Opiates and benzodiazepines also offer excellent cerebral protection but generally have a longer half-life after significant bolus dosing.
5. Etomidate offers an advantage of cerebral protection and better hemodynamic stability.
a. For the hemodynamically stable and volume-replete patient, consider a **barbiturate** versus **propofol.**
b. For the less hemodynamically stable, consider **etomidate.**
6. Obviously, large spikes in CPP due to hypertension or tachycardia are undesirable and may be mitigated during the procedure by titration of short-acting vasoactive agents such as esmolol or labetalol.
7. Ketamine would generally be considered contraindicated because of its tendency to increase BP, raise CPP, and lower seizure threshold.

VI. PATIENTS WITH RESPIRATORY INSUFFICIENCY

A. Examples of this scenario include intubating the failing asthmatic or performing procedural sedation for a patient with chronic obstructive pulmonary disease or restrictive lung disease.

B. Although any sedative agent could be used, *ketamine* offers the unique advantages of:
1. Bronchodilation
2. *Some* maintenance of airway reflexes
3. *Some* maintenance of ventilatory effort except with rapid bolus infusion

C. Disadvantages of ketamine would be:
1. Increased airway secretion
2. Increased incidence of nausea and vomiting
3. These latter issues can be addressed by preprocedure anticholinergic administration and judicious antiemetics use.

BIBLIOGRAPHY

Aronoff G, Berns J, Buer M, et al. *Drug Prescribing in Renal Failure*, 4th ed. American College of Physicians, 1999: 1–20.

Freeman G, Pervemba R. Geriatric pain management: The anesthesiologist's perspective. *Anesthesiol Clin North Am* 2000; 3:123–142.

Stoelting R, Hiller S. *Pharmacology and Physiology in Anesthetic Practice*, 4th ed. Philadelphia: Lippincott Williams & Wilkins, 2006.

Sedation, Analgesia, and Hemodynamic Management of the Intubated/Ventilated Patient

W. James Phillips

I. OVERVIEW

A. Endotracheal intubation is an extraordinarily stimulating and potentially traumatic event. The stimulation and discomfort continue even after the endotracheal tube is correctly placed and secured.

1. Causes of discomfort and anxiety in this patient population include:
a. Preexisting pain from injury or organ damage
b. Restraints, catheters, lines, and taping
c. Stimulation from the endotracheal (ET) tube against the tracheal mucosa
d. Anxiety and fright from the global effect of being on a ventilator
e. Inability to change or vary position
2. Failure to adequately recognize the need for and treat anxiety and pain may cause:
a. Unnecessary patient suffering
b. Hypertension or tachycardia
c. Increased intracranial pressure (ICP)
d. Cardiac ischemia
e. Psychological distress
3. Tools to measure sedation and anxiety, include the Richmond agitation–sedation scale, the Riker agitation–sedation scale, and the Ramsey scale. Regardless of the technique chosen, frequent reassessment with meticulous medication titration is critical. It may also be difficult to determine the relative contribution of AGITATION versus PAIN.

B. One should begin by maximizing nonpharmacologic techniques such as reassessing patient positioning, status of injuries, taping, catheter placement, room lighting, ambient noise, and *ventilator synchronization*. The sequence described next may then be undertaken.

II. MANAGEMENT SEQUENCE

A. Establish a base of sedation–amnesia. Benzodiazepines provide the mainstay of this effort owing to their ability to provide sedation, amnesia, mild muscle relaxation, anxiolysis, and anticonvulsant activity. Choices include:

1. Midazolam (Versed): 0.03 to 0.05 mg/kg every 3 to 5 minutes until adequate sedation. **Note:** These are higher doses than for typical procedural sedation situations because the patient is already intubated

and the airway is secure. This total dose may then be given every 2 to 3 hours. If adequate but short-lived effect, consider an *infusion*:

a. Midazolam 20 mg/100 mL 0.9% NaCl– infused at 0.01 to 0.03 mg/kg per hour

b. Disadvantages

(1) Unpredictable wake-up time in presence of obesity, increased creatinine, low albumin

2. Lorazepam (Ativan): 0.01 to 0.04 mg/kg. Onset time is up to 20 minutes. It has a slower onset than midazolam and has a longer half-life, allowing bolus dosing of every 4 to 6 hours. If inadequate duration, sedation, consider an infusion of 0.005 to 0.01mg/kg per hour.

3. Diazepam: Has been rendered largely obsolete by lorazepam and midazolam. It may exhibit a remarkably prolonged half-life and offers no advantages over the other benzodiazepines. A rule of thumb is half-life in hours = age in years.

4. Diprivan (Propofol): Is inappropriate for bolus (PRN) sedation because of its short half-life and propensity for hemodynamic depression. It is, however, an excellent sedative when administered by infusion with a reasonably rapid wake-up profile. Dose: 25 to 100 µg/kg per minute.

a. Caveats:

(1) Expect some hypotension.

(2) There is no proven analgesic effect.

(3) The lipid emulsion provides some calories.

(4) It provides no amnesia, and small doses of a benzodiazepine may be needed as a supplement.

(5) **Prolonged doses of >60 µg/kg per minute have been associated with rhabdomyolysis, acidosis, and cardiac arrest in children and even some adult cases.**

B. **If a "pure sedative" is inadequate in achieving patient comfort and tranquility, consider proceeding with the addition of an opioid for** *analgesia*. **Opioids may also blunt the hemodynamic response to endotracheal** *intubation*.

1. Typical choices are:

a. Morphine

b. Hydromorphone

c. Fentanyl

2. For the *hemodynamically stable* patient (with a normal creatinine), morphine is an excellent choice. Dose ranges are 0.05 to 0.15 mg/kg every 1 to 4 hours. Half-life is 2 to 3 hours.

a. An infusion of 0.01 to 0.05 mg/kg per hour may be used, but drug accumulation may be a factor.

b. Caveats:

(1) Beware the active metabolite, which is renally excreted.

(2) Modest reductions in systemic vascular resistance (SVR) may occur.

3. For the *hemodynamically unstable* patient (or the patient with renal insufficiency), consider fentanyl versus hydromorphone.
   a. Hydromorphone
      (1) 7 times as potent as morphine
      (2) Bolus dose 0.005 to 0.02 mg/kg
      (3) Half-life = 2 to 3 hours
      (4) Infusion 25–75 µg/kg per hour
   b. Fentanyl
      (1) 80 to 100 times as potent as morphine

Note: *Excellent hemodynamic stability*

    (2) No active metabolites
    (3) Bolus dose 2 to 4 µg/kg
    (4) Infusion 1 to 5 µg/kg per hour

C. Typical combination bolus therapy
Example for a 100-kg patient: Table 13-1.

D. Dexmedetomidine (Precedex) is an imidazoline α_2 central agonist, with primary action at spinal cord adrenergic receptors. One may consider this agent as a sort of "intravenous clonidine."
1. As such, it provides:
a. Sedation without respiratory depressions
b. Analgesia
c. An opioid-sparing effect
d. Moderate dose-dependent reductions in heart rate and blood pressure
2. It has been used as:
a. An intraoperative intravenous anesthetic
b. An intravenous sedative in the intensive care setting
c. An infusion to ameliorate symptoms of opiate and alcohol withdrawal
3. Dosing is a 1-µg/kg bolus slowly over 1 minute followed by an infusion of 0.3 to 0.7 µg/kg per hour titrated to appropriate sedation. There is minimal residual effect and minimal cross-tolerance with opiates.

E. When hemodynamic modulation is required despite seemingly adequate doses of sedative-analgesics, the following agents may be considered:
1. Heart rate control

TABLE 13-1

TYPICAL COMBINATION BOLUS THERAPY: EXAMPLE FOR A 100-KG PATIENT

Sedative	Analgesic
Midazolam 1–3 mg IV every 1–3 hr,	Fentanyl 200–400 µg IV every 1–3 hr,
or	*or*
Lorazepam 1–4 mg IV every 2–6 hr	Morphine 5–10 mg IV every 2–4 hr
	or
	Hydromorphone 0.5–2 mg IV every 2–4 hr

a. Esmolol: 0.1 to 0.5 mg/kg IV every 10 to 15 minutes: β blocker
b. Labetalol: 5 to 20 mg IV every 10 minutes: α/β blocker
c. Hydralazine: 10 to 20 mg IV every 6 hours: arterial dilator
2. Infusion choices include sodium nitroprusside, fenoldopam, and nicardipine

F. Treating agitation: true agitation may be due to psychiatric illness, organic delirium, or intoxication. Benzodiazepines themselves may occasionally cause a paradoxical agitation. In such cases, a legitimate tranquilizer may be useful.
1. Haloperidol (Haldol) is a butyrophenone that has been, perhaps, the most frequently used agent. Typical doses are 2 to 5 mg IV every 20 minutes titrated to effect. One third to one fourth of this effective dose may then be given every 6 to 8 hours.
2. Side effects from Haldol include hypotension and extrapyramidal symptoms. It is sometimes combined with lorazepam in a ratio of 1:5 (mg lorazepam to mg Haldol) to achieve a synergistic calming effect with lower doses of both agents.
3. Droperidol (Inapsine) was an equally effective butyrophenone but is now U.S. Food and Drug Administration (FDA) "black-boxed" off the market owing to accusations of cardiac side effects.
4. Of the antipsychotic agents, olanzapine (Zyprexa) is also a very reasonable choice because of its minimal sedative effect and decreased incidence of extrapyramidal effects. Dose is 10 mg IM titrated every 2 to 3 hours to a maximum of 30 mg/day.

III. FINAL CAVEATS

A. Benzodiazepines are excellent first choices for sedating intubated patients.

B. Remember that being intubated and ventilated may be very uncomfortable, making assessing sites and severity of pain difficult.

C. Opiates are excellent adjuncts to the benzodiazepines or Diprivan.

D. Fentanyl is an excellent analgesic in the hemodynamically unstable patient or in the presence of renal insufficiency.

E. Opiate: benzodiazepine co-administration provides an excellent synergistic mix, but the side effects of hypotension, respiratory depression, and longer wake-up times may be significant.

F. Careful assessment, drug titration, and reassessment are the keys to success.

G. If PRN doses need to be given too frequently, consider an infusion. Good infusion choices include propofol, fentanyl, and midazolam > lorazepam.

Providing Comfort at the End of Life

W. James Phillips

I. PHARMACOLOGIC SYMPTOM MANAGEMENT

A. Introduction

1. There will come a phase of care for all patients during which the practitioner must shift from a cure to a care focus. Regardless of the baseline diagnosis, the situation must eventually evolve to one in which symptom management tightly interwoven with meeting the emotional needs of the patient becomes the order of the day.
2. Such palliative care will not be confined to those patients with terminal metastatic cancer. Recent data indicate that although cancer remains the predominant diagnosis in hospice programs (46%), there has been a significant growth in diagnoses related to other organ system derangements.
3. This chapter cannot be a comprehensive review of an extraordinarily complex area. Indeed, the services of an entire palliative care team, particularly for care in the home setting, may be required. This team may include:
   a. Core attending physicians
   b. Registered nurse
   c. Social worker
   d. Chaplain
   e. Pharmacist
   f. Physical therapist
   g. Volunteers
   h. Key family members
4. Critical duties of this team include, but are not limited to:
   a. Arrival at a firm and conclusive diagnosis utilizing consultations and necessary testing.
   b. Articulation of a rational and reasonable care plan with appropriate expectations.
   c. Clear and compassionate **communication** of this plan to the patient and family.
   d. Execution of the plan **with the patient and family.**
   e. Frequent and timely reassessments.
   f. Balancing unrealistic expectations with the need to **constantly watch** for reversible causes of deterioration (e.g., infection, dehydration, pathologic fractures needing stabilization).
   g. Understanding that embarking on a course of palliative care **is** *not* **giving up; it is** *aggressively* **directing the care plan in a new direction.**

h. **Believing that the efforts and emotions expended making a patient's end time tolerable if not comfortable are as important as any other medical interventions in the course of a life.**

B. Terminal diagnoses

1. Diagnoses encountered that may necessitate the institution of a palliative care plan, if not formal hospice program referral, may include:
a. Cancer: widely metastatic or inoperable
b. Cardiac disease: congestive heart failure with symptoms at rest or inoperable coronary disease with class IV angina
c. Pulmonary disease: end-stage obstructive or restrictive disease not amenable to transplantation
   (1) Forced expiratory volume < 30%
   (2) Hypoxemia despite oxygen
   (3) Chronic CO_2 retention with right heart failure
d. Renal disease: renal failure not amenable to transplantation or dialysis
e. Neurologic disease: severe cognitive impairment, severe poststroke motor impairment with decubitus, or recurrent aspiration
f. Infectious diseases: end-stage acquired immunodeficiency syndrome (AIDS)
2. It is critical to appreciate that regardless of the diagnosis, attention must be paid not only to *physical symptoms* but also to the *emotional*, *affective*, *sensory*, and *functional* impact of the disease on the patient and family. Compassionate acknowledgment of the family caregivers in relation to the patient will enhance caregiving ability and patient care. Although this chapter focuses on pharmacologic symptom management, many nonpharmacologic interventions are available that may prove efficacious.
3. Specific symptoms that will be addressed are:
a. Pain
b. Distress and anxiety
c. Shortness of breath
d. Fatigue
e. Nausea and vomiting
f. Constipation
g. Anorexia
h. Insomnia

C. Pain

1. Pain is likely to accompany any terminal illness. Examples include bony pain from metastases, neurogenic pain from ischemia or chemotherapy-induced neuropathy, or intractable visceral pain from cardiac ischemic or pancreatic carcinoma. These represent examples of musculoskeletal pain, neuropathic pain, and visceral pain, respectively. Although opiates will be the foundation for treatment of all these entities, certain adjuvant agents may be selectively useful in specific cases.

2. Some caveats of successful opiate therapy are:

a. Intermittent pain may be successfully treated with short-acting, immediate-release agents such as Tylenol with codeine, Tylenol with oxycodone (Percocet, Tylox), Tylenol with hydrocodone (Lortab), morphine sulfate immediate release (MSIR), and oxycodone immediate release (Roxicodone).

b. More severe or constant pain requires:
   (1) A long-acting agent for sustained blood levels
       (a) MS Contin every 12 hr ("Avinza" and "Kadian" preparations may give 24-hour duration analgesia)
       (b) OxyContin every 12 hr
       (c) Methadone every 12 hr

Note: *Fentanyl patch is changed every 48 to 72 hours (blood levels require 15 to 24 hours, so poor choice for changing pain levels).*

   (2) Combine with a short-acting agent for breakthrough pain, such as MS Contin, 30 to 60 mg every 12 hours, **with** MSIR, 30 mg every 4 to 6 hours PRN, or Tylenol with oxycodone, 5 to 10 mg every 4 to 6 hours PRN.

c. Initiate laxative therapy whenever a long-acting opiate is started (see Constipation).

d. Initiate PRN antiemetic agents whenever a long-acting opiate is started (see Nausea and Vomiting).

e. Reassure patients that addiction is **rare.**
   (1) If current agents fail, others are available.
   (2) Pain should not be under-reported.

f. Titrate opiates until analgesia is obtained or side effects are limiting. Frequent surveillance is needed. Maximize use of opiate rotation and alternative routes of delivery.

g. There is no role for mixed agonists-antagonists or partial agonists because of the ceiling effect and potential for reversing the effect of previous or planned pure agonists.

h. Agents **to be avoided** include:
   (1) Propoxyphene: potential toxicity, lack of efficacy
   (2) Meperidine: active metabolite, significant euphoria, short half-life

i. Maximize alternative routes of delivery.
   (1) Transdermal in cases of dysphagia.
   (2) Subcutaneous or transmucosal for severe pain flares.
   (3) Tunneled epidural catheters when other routes and modalities have been exhausted.

j. Maximize use of adjuvant analgesics.

k. Maximize use of **adjuvant techniques** (Table 14-1) such as radiation therapy for bone pain, localized tumors, and central nervous system (CNS) or spinal tumors (beware delayed cognitive decline). Brachytherapy or systemic radionucleotides (e.g., strontium) may also provide significant benefit.

TABLE 14-1

ADJUVANTS

Agent	Dose	Indication
Prednisone	10–40 mg every day	Bone pain Neuropathic pain including spinal cord compressions
Dexamethasone	4–20 mg every day daily	Same as above
Gabapentin	300–900 mg 3 times	Neuropathic pain
(Tegretol, Dilantin, baclofen may be substituted but have more toxicity and side effects and no greater demonstrated efficacy)	Start 100–300 mg 3 times daily Advance 300 mg every 3 days Adjust for increased creatinine	
Amitriptyline	10–150 every night Start 10–25 mg at bedtime Advance 25 mg every 3–5 days Beware anticholinergic effects! Nortriptyline perhaps recommended for age > 60 yr (fewer anticholinergic effects)	Neuropathic pain Musculoskeletal pain
Bisphosphonates	Variable Available PO, IV	Bone metastases
Various esoteric IV regimens	Phentolamine	Neuropathic, visceral pain
	Dexmedetomidine	Neuropathic pain
	Octreotide	Visceral abdominal pain
	Lidocaine	Neuropathic pain

D. Anxiety, depression, and distress

1. It will be difficult to separate out these entities. Although a number of screening tools may be available, *one should consider simply asking the patient if he or she feels depressed.*
2. It is also imperative to try and separate the *components* of *anxiety* and *depression* because pharmacologic management will vary tremendously. It will also be critical to assess any component of delirium or agitation because tranquilizing or antipsychotic agents may be necessary.
3. Depression caveats:
a. If significant pain is present, the tricyclic agents have a much greater demonstrated analgesic effect than the selective serotonin reuptake inhibitors (SSRIs).

b. The SSRIs have a much more favorable side-effect profile than the tricyclics, particularly related to anticholinergic effects.

c. Psychostimulants may be potentially useful as antidepressants and co-analgesics (methylphenidate and dextroamphetamine).

4. Anxiolysis caveats:

a. Lorazepam, diazepam, and clonazepam may all be useful. Beware the markedly prolonged half-life of diazepam with advancing age. Midazolam might be the drug of choice for IV or SC use.

b. Starting doses

    (1) Lorazepam 1 to 2 mg PO every 6 hours

    (2) Diazepam 2.5 to 5 mg PO every 6 to 8 hours

    (3) Clonazepam 0.5 mg PO every 8 hours

5. Agitation and delirium caveats

Historically, haloperidol, 2 to 4 mg PO every 6 to 8 hours, has been a mainstay. Newer antipsychotics such as olanzapine and risperidone have fewer extrapyramidal side effects. Each of these agents is also available as an orally disintegrating tablet. The latter is also available in liquid form.

E. Shortness of breath

1. It is critical to rule out reversible causes of dyspnea:

a. Pleural effusion → withdraw fluid

b. Pericardial effusion → withdraw fluid

c. Progressive anemia → transfuse

d. Pneumonia → antibiotics, oxygen

e. Chronic obstructive pulmonary disease or asthma exacerbation → steroids, bronchodilators, oxygen

f. Angina → nitroglycerin, oxygen, analgesics, transfuse (?)

g. Fluid overload → furosemide PO or IV, nitroglycerin sublingually or transdermally, oxygen

h. Acidosis → correction of underlying cause

i. Excessive secretions → transdermal scopolamine, IV glycopyrrolate 0.2 mg every 4 to 6 hours

j. Anxiety → anxiolytics

2. When reversible causes have been addressed, cough suppressants may be useful:

a. Guaifenesin 100 to 400 mg PO every 4 to 6 hours

b. Dextromethorphan 10 to 20 mg PO every 4 to 6 hours

Note: *Nebulized morphine, 0.2 to 0.3 mg/kg, may relieve dyspnea in terminal cancer cases.*

F. Fatigue

1. This is an inevitable symptom that may be due to cardiac or pulmonary dysfunction, burden of disease, electrolyte or muscle abnormalities,

endocrine changes, thyroid adrenal, or anemia. When these indices have been optimized, the following agents may be considered:
a. Epoetin (Epogen) SC 3 times weekly—onset 2 to 3 weeks (may be useful to cancer-related fatigue even if anemia modest)
b. Stimulants
   (1) Methylphenidate 2.5 to 10 mg every morning or noon (available as sustained release)
   (2) Dextroamphetamine 2.5 to 10 mg every morning or noon
   (3) Modafinil 100 to 200 mg PO every morning (minimal heart rate, blood pressure changes)
c. Corticosteroids: variable doses enhance appetite and sense of well-being.

G. Nausea and vomiting
1. This symptom may be initiated at sites ranging from the gastrointestinal tract to the inner ear, midbrain, and cerebral cortex.
2. Gastrointestinal causes include:
a. Reflux → antacids
b. Ileus → motility agents
c. Abdominal masses → corticosteroids anticholinergics
3. Inner ear causes include:
a. Movement
   (1) Antihistamines
   (2) Meclizine
   (3) Sedatives (diazepam)
   (4) Anticholinergics (scopolamine)
b. Inner ear dysfunction
   (1) Decongestants
   (2) Antihistamines
4. Midbrain or chemoreceptor trigger zone causes include:
a. Electrolyte imbalance → increased calcium, sodium derangement
b. Drug effect (opiates) → add antiemetics
c. Cerebral metastases → corticosteroids, antiemetics
5. Cortical causes include:
a. Anxiety → anxiolytic
b. Pain → analgesic
6. A summary of drug choices is given in Table 14-2.

H. Constipation
1. The most common causes of this symptom are likely opiate treatment and dehydration and electrolyte disorders. Primary bowel issues such as obstruction or ileus also need to be ruled out.
2. In the absence of organic disease, the agents listed in Table 14-3 may be useful.

TABLE 14-2

SUMMARY OF DRUGS THAT CAN BE USED TO ALLEVIATE NAUSEA AND VOMITING

Mechanism	Agent	Dose	Caveats
Dopamine antagonists	Promethazine (Phenergan)	12.5–25 mg IV or Po q 6–8°	Also antihistamine available as suppository
	Prochlorperazine (Compazine) (Droperidol-great drug "Black-boxed" out of use. Complain to U.S. Food and Drug Administration)	5–10 mg IV or Po q 6–8°	Available as suppository
Antihistamines	Diphenhydramine (Benadryl)	25 mg IV/PO every 8 hr	
	Hydroxyzine (Vistaril)	25–50 mg IM every 8 hr	Not advised IV
Anticholinergics	Scopolamine patch (1.5 mg)	Every 72 hr (4 hr onset)	Beware central anticholinergic syndrome in elderly
	Glycopyrrolate (Robinul)	0.2 mg IV every 6 hr	
Serotonin antagonists	Ondansetron (Zofran)	4–8 mg PO every 8 hr	Expensive
	Granisetron (Kytril)	1 mg PO twice daily	Expensive
	Dolasetron (Anzemet)	1.8 mg/kg PO/IV	Expensive

TABLE 14-3

AGENTS THAT MAY BE USED TO ALLEVIATE CONSTIPATION

Agent	Action	Dose
Bisacodyl (Dulcolax)	Stimulant	5 mg PO daily
Senna (Senokot)	Stimulant and increased peristalsis	2 tablets once or twice daily
Docusate (Colace)	Stool softener fat dissolution	1–2 tablets twice daily
Magnesium hydroxide (milk of magnesium)	Osmotic	30 mL PO three times daily
Magnesium citrate	Osmotic	240 mL PO daily
Lactulose	Osmotic	30 mL PO three times daily
Castor oil	Osmotic	15–30 mL PO

I. Anorexia

1. Reversible causes of anorexia include:
a. Hypercalcemia
b. Hypernatremia or hyponatremia
c. Hypothyroidism
d. Infection
e. Adrenal insufficiency
f. Gastrointestinal motility disorders
g. Uncontrolled diabetes
h. Congestive heart failure
i. Oral thrush
j. Reflux
k. Esophagitis
2. When reversible causes have been addressed, the following agents may be useful for appetite stimulation:
a. Various antiemetics
b. Megestrol acetate (Megace) 100 to 200 mg PO four times daily
c. Prednisone (negative effect on muscle mass)
d. Dexamethasone
e. Dronabinol (Marinol) 2.5 to 5 mg PO three times daily; also antiemetic; expensive

J. Insomnia

1. Before initiating an analgesic regimen strictly for sleep, it is imperative that:
a. Pain is controlled.
b. Depression and anxiety are addressed.
2. To this end, one should consider:
a. Initiating or titrating a long-acting opiate each evening, such as:
   (1) MS Contin
   (2) OxyContin
   (3) Methadone
b. Initiating or titrating a tricyclic antidepressant, such as

(1) Amitriptyline (Elavil)

(2) Nortriptyline (Pamelor)

c. Both are excellent **sleep aids** and **co-analgesics.**

3. If these are ineffective or not indicated the following agents may be useful:

a. Diphenhydramine (Benadryl): 25 to 50 mg PO at bedtime

b. Hydroxyzine (Vistaril): 25 to 50 mg PO at bedtime

c. Zolpidem (Ambien): 5 to 10 mg PO at bedtime

d. Zaleplon (Sonata): 5 to 10 mg PO at bedtime

e. Clonazepam (Klonopin): 0.5 to 2 mg PO at bedtime

II. FINAL CAVEATS

A. Palliative care does not mean you are quitting!

B. The search and surveillance for reversible causes of deterioration or increased symptoms must be relentless.

C. Pain, distress, anxiety, and depression must all be aggressively addressed.

D. Communication and meticulous attention to the emotional needs of the patient and family are paramount.

BIBLIOGRAPHY

de Leon-Casasola O. *Cancer Pain: Pharmacological, Interventional and Palliative Care Approaches*. Philadelphia: WB Saunders, 2006.

Lipman A, Jackson I, Tyler L. *Evidence Based Symptom Control in Palliative Care: Systemic Reviews and Validated Clinical Practice Guidelines for 15 Common Problems in Patients with Life Limiting Disease*. Salt Lake City: Haworth Press, 2000.

Watson M, Lucas C, Hoy A, Back I. *Oxford Handbook of Palliative Care*. Oxford, UK: Oxford University Press, 2005.

Appendix A: UMC Sedation Policy

The University Hospitals and Clinics
The University of Mississippi Medical Center
Jackson, Mississippi

**HOSPITAL ADMINISTRATIVE POLICY AND
PROCEDURE MANUAL**

Subject: Procedural Sedation

Effective Date: 7/02
Review/Revision Date: 9/02, 11/04, 1/05, 4/05, 4/06
Prepared by: Procedural Sedation Policy and Procedure Committee

I. PURPOSE:

University of Mississippi Medical Center will provide an environment for safe and effective sedation for diagnostic, therapeutic, and invasive procedures. Patient safety and comfort are top priorities, and a high level of readiness for emergency situations is necessary in all cases and in all areas of the hospital where sedation is used.

Moderate sedation/analgesia and deep sedation/analgesia for diagnostic, therapeutic, and invasive procedures shall be practiced throughout the hospital in accordance with the following guidelines. Departmental policies will be developed to meet special needs of unique patient populations, which shall meet or exceed the personnel and monitoring guidelines described herein. This policy covers nonanesthesiology staff physicians, dentists, residents, nurse practitioners, and/or registered nurses.

A. Definitions:

These definitions identify levels of sedation in a continuum from minimal sedation to general anesthesia.

1. <u>Minimal sedation (anxiolysis)</u>—a medically induced state during which patients respond normally to verbal commands. Cognitive function and coordination may be impaired; ventilatory and cardiovascular systems are unaffected.
2. <u>Moderate sedation/analgesia</u> ("conscious sedation")—a drug-induced depression of consciousness during which patients respond purposefully to verbal commands, either alone or accompanied by light tactile stimulation. No interventions are required to maintain a patent airway, and spontaneous ventilation is adequate. Cardiovascular function is usually maintained.
3. <u>Deep sedation/analgesia</u>—a drug-induced depression of consciousness during which patients cannot easily be aroused but respond

purposefully following repeated or painful stimulation. The ability to independently maintain ventilatory function may be impaired. Patients undergoing deep sedation have a significant risk for partial or complete loss of protective reflexes, including the ability to consistently maintain a patent airway independently and the inability to respond purposefully to physical stimulation or verbal commands. Loss of gag reflex, inability to handle oral secretions, and loss of swallowing reflex may occur. Patients may require assistance in maintaining a patent airway, and spontaneous ventilation may be inadequate. Cardiovascular function is usually maintained.

4. <u>Anesthesia</u>—consists of general anesthesia and spinal or major regional anesthesia. It does not include local anesthesia. General anesthesia is a drug-induced loss of consciousness during which patients are not arousable, even by painful stimulation. The ability to independently maintain ventilatory function is often impaired. Patients often require assistance in maintaining a patent airway, and positive pressure ventilation may be required because of depressed spontaneous ventilation or drug-induced depression of neuromuscular function. Cardiovascular function may be impaired.

II. SCOPE:

A. This policy applies to the use of moderate sedation/analgesia and deep sedation/analgesia in all hospital departments and areas that are non OR or Anesthesia.

B. This policy does not cover patients who are mechanically ventilated receiving sedation or patients receiving anxiolytic or analgesic agents, which are administered routinely to alleviate pain and agitation (e.g., sedation for treatment of insomnia, sedatives for anxiety disorders, preoperative medications for surgery, postoperative analgesia, analgesia for chronic pain conditions, pain control during labor and delivery).

III. POLICY:

A. The departmental chairman and/or manager shall be responsible for ensuring that the standards outlined in this general policy are met or exceeded for the department's practice.

B. The department chairman and/or manager will be responsible for maintaining and updating credentialing/privileges for Procedural Sedation initially and on the practitioner's reappointment cycle and will ensure that the most current information is maintained on the UMC physician credentialing and resident/fellow privileging website.

1. Application of Delineation of Clinical or Practice Privileges for Procedural Sedation will be completed by the requesting practitioner, including the supporting documentation.

2. The Department Chairman will review and approve the requested privileges and attest that the practitioner is competent.

3. The Credentials Committee will review and grant approval of the privileges.
4. The Medical Executive Committee will review and grant final approval of the privileges.

C. Procedural Sedation privileges/credentialing for staff physicians, dentists, residents, and nurse practitioners will require meeting one criterion from each section below:
1. Section 1
a. Completion of training in clinical subspecialty that provides training in Procedural Sedation.
b. Completion of specialty/fellowship training that included a rotation in Anesthesia/Critical Care.
c. Completion of credentialing board requirements for advanced clinical practicum and completion of certification examination in Acute Care. (nurse practitioners only)
2. Section 2
a. Successful completion of the UMC web-based Procedural Sedation Course/Exam. This exam must be passed every 2 years. (residents/nurse practitioners only)
b. Attendance/participation in a UMC Approved Procedural Sedation Training program. (physicians and dentists only)
c. Provision of a good-faith estimate of the number of instances of each type of procedure in which sedation is administered with a list of any adverse events related to the sedation during those cases, including causal analysis, treatment, and outcome. (physicians and dentists only)
3. Section 3
a. Current ACLS, PALS, and/or NRP as appropriate to the patient population.
b. Board Certified in Anesthesiology, Emergency Medicine, Interventional or Critical Care Specialties that include Procedural Sedation in the clinical training program.
c. Other Board Certifications that include Procedural Sedation in the clinical training program and the use of vasoactive medications and airway management on a routine basis.

D. Procedural Sedation privileges for residents will require meeting the following additional requirements as outlined below:
1. PGY 2 or above.
2. Each procedure/patient will be discussed with the faculty of record prior to commencement of the procedure.

E. Procedural Sedation privileges for nurse practitioners will require the following additional requirements as outlined below:
1. Procedure being performed by the nurse practitioner must be within the scope of practice according to the National Scope of Practice guidelines.

2. Controlled Substance Prescriptive Authority Schedule II–V approval from the Mississippi Board of Nursing.
3. Each procedure/patient will be discussed with the faculty of record prior to commencement of the procedure.

F. The registered nurse monitoring the patient will require the following specific training process:

1. Attend the orientation course with successful completion as evidenced by a passing score of 80% or greater on the exam and complete the competency checklist.
2. Achieve competency in EKG monitoring by successfully completing the Basic EKG class or successfully challenging the examination and maintain competency on an annual basis according to the EKG Competency Policy NADM/E-2.
3. Current ACLS, PALS, NRP as appropriate to the patient population.
4. The department manager is responsible for maintaining employee's education and competency on file. The employee's file will be updated on an annual basis.

G. All sedation will be ordered and supervised by an appropriately credentialed/privileged physician, dentist, resident, or nurse practitioner trained in professional standards and techniques to administer pharmacologic agents to achieve desired levels of sedation and to monitor patients carefully in order to maintain them at the desired level of sedation.

H. Minimum personnel during the sedation process shall be two qualified professionals with one patient. One is the qualified practitioner who directs the sedation and may be performing the procedure. The second is a qualified registered nurse or practitioner whose only responsibility is the constant observation and monitoring of the patient and the necessary documentation. Observation and monitoring will be done from the start of sedation until discharge criteria have been met.

IV. EQUIPMENT:

Appropriate to the Adult, Pediatric, and/or Neonatal patient.

A. At the bedside

   Suction and suction catheters
   Positive pressure breathing device
   Oxygen and delivery devices (nasal, cannula, face mask)
   Appropriate-size oral airways
   Cardiac monitor, blood pressure measuring apparatus
   Pulse oximeter
   Reversal agents naloxone (Narcan) and flumazenil (Romazicon)
   IV supplies

B. Readily available
>Emergency cart
>Defibrillator

V. PROCEDURE:

A. Preprocedure documentation should be recorded on the Procedural Sedation Record, to include the following:

1. A history will be performed by the registered nurse and/or the practitioner and should include the following:
a. Medical history
b. Current medications
c. Social history
d. Adverse reactions (medications, food, latex)
e. Weight in pounds and kilograms of all pediatric and neonatal patients
2. The practitioner or registered nurse will verify the patient, procedure, and/or site/side against the consent form. Refer to policy HADM/S-4.
3. The presedation physical assessment will be completed by the performing practitioner, which will include the following (residents and nurse practitioners will discuss the assessment with the faculty of record prior to the commencement of Procedural Sedation):
a. Document the need for sedation
b. Patient's physical assessment
c. Plan of care for the patient
d. Assign an Aldrete score
e. Assign the ASA score
f. Obtain an informed consent for procedural sedation from the patient, guardian and/or family/responsible adult prior to the administration of analgesia. If an emergent circumstance exists; then implied consent is given.
g. Evaluate the appropriate preprocedure labs, x-rays, and EKG, including a pregnancy test, if applicable.
h. Verify that all outpatients have appropriate transportation.
4. Intravenous access will be initiated as indicated below:
a. Planned IV sedation
b. As determination by the practitioner
c. Any patient with an ASA of III or greater, even if receiving PO sedation
5. NPO status will be documented as follows:
a. No solids, 8 hours prior to procedure
b. No full liquids, 6 hours prior to procedure
c. No clear liquids, 2 hours prior to procedure
d. Times should not be modified unless thoroughly documented that the procedure must be done on an emergency basis. If this patient experiences deep sedation, the patient must be intubated to protect the airway.
6. Patient education should be documented on the patient education form or in the nurse's notes.

B. Intraprocedure documentation should include:
1. The presedation assessment will be completed no more than 5 minutes before initial administration of analgesia/sedation.
a. Verify patient, procedure, site, and availability of equipment. Refer to policy HADM/S-4.
b. Pain assessment
c. Vital signs: Blood pressure, heart rate, and respiratory rate
d. EKG rhythm
e. O_2 saturation
f. Airway patency
g. Supplemental O_2 will be provided unless contraindicated. Suggested rate of administration is adults, 2 L/minute per nasal cannula, and pediatrics, the same or 40% blow-by.
h. Level of consciousness
i. Temperature
j. Medications given; note medication, route, dose, and initial of person administering medication. The Procedural Sedation Drug Table contains the recommended dosing for moderate and deep sedation for adult and pediatric patients as a guide for the practitioners and registered nurses.
2. Assessment will be documented every 5 minutes at a minimum once the first analgesia/sedation has been administered:
a. Vital signs: blood pressure, heart rate, and respiratory rate
b. EKG rhythm
c. O_2 saturation
d. Airway patency
e. Supplemental O_2
f. Level of consciousness
g. Pain
h. Medications given; note medication, route, dose, and initial of person administering medication.

C. Adverse drug reaction form must be completed if an adverse drug reaction occurs or if a reversal agent is administered.

D. Postprocedure documentation should include:
1. RN monitoring patient may be responsible for up to a maximum of two patients.
2. Assessment is documented every 15 minutes times 4, then every 30 minutes times 2, then hourly or until the discharge criteria have been met.
a. Vital signs: Blood pressure, heart rate, and respiratory rate
b. EKG rhythm
c. O_2 saturation
d. Airway patency
e. Supplemental O_2
f. Level of consciousness
g. Pain score

h. Temperature (once if normal)
3. If the patient receives a reversal agent, the patient will observed post procedure for a minimum of 1.5 additional hours.
4. If the patient requires transfer prior to meeting discharge criteria, the patient will be transferred to the appropriate area with a qualified RN and/or practitioner to continue continuous monitoring.

E. Patients may be transferred to an inpatient unit, ambulatory surgery unit, or to a registered nurse and/or licensed practical nurse with a full patient load once the following inpatient discharge criteria have been met.
1. Vital signs: blood pressure, heart rate and respiratory rate within 20% of normal or at presedation value
2. EKG rhythm normal or at presedation rhythm
3. O_2 saturation normal or at presedation value
4. Airway is patent.
5. Level of consciousness within 20% of normal or presedation value
6. Pain score at or below 4
7. Temperature > 97° F/36.1° C or below 100° F/37.7° C
8. Postsedation Aldrete score within 20% of presedation score

F. Patients may be discharged home after first meeting the inpatient discharge criteria and then meeting the following outpatient discharge criteria:
1. No sign or symptoms that may jeopardize the safety of recovery (i.e., bleeding, swelling, extreme pain, excessive nausea and vomiting, or dizziness).
2. Discharge orders written.
3. Discharge planning has been reviewed with patient, family/accompanying responsible adult as appropriate; provide written home care instruction.
4. Provide follow-up for extended care as indicated. Next day follow-up phone call is recommended to evaluate status.
5. Provide 24-hour call-back number.
6. Ensure that the patient's belongings are returned and that their return is documented.

G. Units responsible for monitoring and management of patients receiving sedation will complete a Performance Improvement Monitor for each patient receiving procedural sedation. The monitor form will be sent to the Department of Performance Improvement on a monthly basis. The performance improvement will collect data for analysis by the Procedural Sedation Committee.

H. Sedation practices throughout the University Hospitals and Clinics shall be monitored and evaluated by the Department of Anesthesiology according to the policy as outlined.

Appendix B: DEA Drug Schedule Overview

TITLE 21—FOOD AND DRUGS; CHAPTER 13—DRUG ABUSE PREVENTION AND CONTROL; SUBCHAPTER I—CONTROL AND ENFORCEMENT; PART B—AUTHORITY TO CONTROL; STANDARDS AND SCHEDULES; SEC. 812. SCHEDULES OF CONTROLLED SUBSTANCES

Statute

(a) Establishment: There are established five schedules of controlled substances, to be known as schedules I, II, III, IV, and V. Such schedules shall initially consist of the substances listed in this section. The schedules established by this section shall be updated and republished on a semiannual basis during the 2-year period beginning 1 year after October 27, 1970, and shall be updated and republished on an annual basis thereafter.

(b) Placement on schedules; findings required: Except where control is required by United States obligations under an international treaty, convention, or protocol, in effect on October 27, 1970, and except in the case of an immediate precursor, a drug or other substance may not be placed in any schedule unless the findings required for such schedule are made with respect to such drug or other substance. The findings required for each of the schedules are as follows:

(1) Schedule I.
(A) The drug or other substance has a high potential for abuse.
(B) The drug or other substance has no currently accepted medical use in treatment in the United States.
(C) There is a lack of accepted safety for use of the drug or other substance under medical supervision.
(2) Schedule II.
(A) The drug or other substance has a high potential for abuse.
(B) The drug or other substance has a currently accepted medical use in treatment in the United States or a currently accepted medical use with severe restrictions.
(C) Abuse of the drug or other substances may lead to severe psychological or physical dependence.
(3) Schedule III.
(A) The drug or other substance has a potential for abuse less than the drugs or other substances in schedules I and II.
(B) The drug or other substance has a currently accepted medical use in treatment in the United States.
(C) Abuse of the drug or other substance may lead to moderate or low physical dependence or high psychological dependence.

(4) Schedule IV.

(A) The drug or other substance has a low potential for abuse relative to the drugs or other substances in schedule III.

(B) The drug or other substance has a currently accepted medical use in treatment in the United States.

(C) Abuse of the drug or other substance may lead to limited physical dependence or psychological dependence relative to the drugs or other substances in schedule III.

(5) Schedule V.

(A) The drug or other substance has a low potential for abuse relative to the drugs or other substances in schedule IV.

(B) The drug or other substance has a currently accepted medical use in treatment in the United States.

(C) Abuse of the drug or other substance may lead to limited physical dependence or psychological dependence relative to the drugs or other substances in schedule IV.

(c) Initial schedules of controlled substances Schedules I, II, III, IV, and V shall, unless and until amended pursuant to section 811 of this title, consist of the following drugs or other substances, by whatever official name, common or usual name, chemical name, or brand name designated: Revised schedules are published in the Code of Federal Regulations, Part 1308 of Title 21, Food and Drugs.

U.S. Drug Enforcement Administration (DEA): Title 21, Section 812. Available at http://www.usdoj.gov/dea/pubs/csa/812.htm.

Appendix C: DEA Drug Scheduling

This document is a general reference and not a comprehensive list. This list describes the basic or parent chemical and does not describe the salts, isomers and salts of isomers, esters, ethers, and derivatives that may also be controlled substances.

<u>SCHEDULE I</u>

Substance	DEA Number	Non-narcotic	Other Names
1-(1-Phenylcyclohexyl)pyrrolidine	7458	N	PCPy, PHP, rolicyclidine
1-(2-Phenylethyl)-4-phenyl-4-acetoxypiperidine	9663		PEPAP, synthetic heroin
1-[1-(2-Thienyl)cyclohexyl]piperidine	7470	N	TCP, tenocyclidine
1-[1-(2-Thienyl)cyclohexyl]pyrrolidine	7473	N	TCPy
1-Methyl-4-phenyl-4-propionoxypiperidine	9661		MPPP, synthetic heroin
2,5-Dimethoxy-4-ethylamphetamine	7399	N	DOET
2,5-Dimethoxyamphetamine	7396	N	DMA, 2,5-DMA
3,4,5-Trimethoxyamphetamine	7390	N	TMA
3,4-Methylenedioxyamphetamine	7400	N	MDA, Love Drug
3,4-Methylenedioxymethamphetamine	7405	N	MDMA, Ecstasy, XTC
3,4-Methylenedioxy-N-ethylamphetamine	7404	N	N-ethyl MDA, MDE, MDEA
3-Methylfentanyl	9813		China White, fentanyl
3-Methylthiofentanyl	9833		Chine White, fentanyl
4-Bromo-2,5-dimethoxyamphetamine	7391	N	DOB, 4-bromo-DMA
4-Bromo-2,5-dimethoxyphenethylamine	7392	N	Nexus, 2-CB, has been sold as Ecstasy, i.e., MDMA
4-Methoxyamphetamine	7411	N	PMA
4-Methyl-2,5-dimethoxyamphetamine	7395	N	DOM, STP
4-Methylaminorex (cis isomer)	1590	N	U4Euh, McN-422
5-Methoxy-3,4-methylenedioxyamphetamine	7401	N	MMDA
Acetorphine	9319		
Acetyl-alpha-methylfentanyl	9815		
Acetyldihydrocodeine	9051		Acetylcodone
Acetylmethadol	9601		Methadyl acetate
Allylprodine	9602		
Alphacetylmethadol except levo-alphacetylmethadol	9603		
Alpha-Ethyltryptamine	7249	N	ET, Trip
Alphameprodine	9604		
Alphamethadol	9605		
Alpha-Methylfentanyl	9814		China White, fentanyl

SCHEDULE I—CONT'D

Substance	DEA Number	Non-narcotic	Other Names
Alpha-Methylthiofentanyl	9832		China White, fentanyl
Aminorex	1585	N	has been sold as methamphetamine
Benzethidine	9606		
Benzylmorphine	9052		
Betacetylmethadol	9607		
Beta-Hydroxy-3-methylfentanyl	9831		China White, fentanyl
Beta-Hydroxyfentanyl	9830		China White, fentanyl
Betameprodine	9608		
Betamethadol	9609		
Betaprodine	9611		
Bufotenine	7433	N	Mappine, N,N-dimethylserotonin
Cathinone	1235	N	Constituent of Khat plant
Clonitazene	9612		
Codeine methylbromide	9070		
Codeine-N-oxide	9053		
Cyprenorphine	9054		
Desomorphine	9055		
Dextromoramide	9613		Palfium, Jetrium, Narcolo
Diampromide	9615		
Diethylthiambutene	9616		
Diethyltryptamine	7434	N	DET
Difenoxin	9168		Lyspafen
Dihydromorphine	9145		
Dimenoxadol	9617		
Dimepheptanol	9618		
Dimethylthiambutene	9619		
Dimethyltryptamine	7435	N	DMT
Dioxaphetyl butyrate	9621		
Dipipanone	9622		Dipipan, phenylpiperone HCl, Diconal, Wellconal
Drotebanol	9335		Metebanyl, oxymethebanol
Ethylmethylthiambutene	9623		
Etonitazene	9624		
Etorphine (except HCl)	9056		
Etoxeridine	9625		
Fenethylline	1503	N	Captagon, amfetyline, ethyltheophylline amphetamine
Furethidine	9626		
Gamma-Hydroxybutyric acid (GHB)	2010	N	GHB, gamma-hydroxybutyrate, sodium oxybate
Heroin	9200		Diacetylmorphine, diamorphine
Hydromorphinol	9301		
Hydroxypethidine	9627		
Ibogaine	7260	N	Constituent of Tabernanthe iboga plant

(Continued)

DEA DRUG SCHEDULING

SCHEDULE I—CONT'D

Substance	DEA Number	Non-narcotic	Other Names
Ketobemidone	9628		Cliradon
Levomoramide	9629		
Levophenacylmorphan	9631		
Lysergic acid diethylamide	7315	N	LSD, lysergide
Marijuana	7360	N	Cannabis, marijuana
Mecloqualone	2572	N	Nubarene
Mescaline	7381	N	Constituent of Peyote cacti
Methaqualone	2565	N	Quaalude, Parest, Somnafac, Opitimil, Mandrax
Methcathinone	1237	N	N-Methylcathinone, "cat"
Methyldesorphine	9302		
Methyldihydromorphine	9304		
Morpheridine	9632		
Morphine methylbromide	9305		
Morphine methylsulfonate	9306		
Morphine-N-oxide	9307		
Myrophine	9308		
N,N-Dimethylamphetamine	1480	N	
N-Ethyl-1-phenylcyclohexylamine	7455	N	PCE
N-Ethyl-3-piperidyl benzilate	7482	N	JB 323
N-Ethylamphetamine	1475	N	NEA
N-Hydroxy-3,4-methylenedioxyamphetamine	7402	N	N-hydroxy MDA
Nicocodeine	9309		
Nicomorphine	9312		Vilan
N-Methyl-3-piperidyl benzilate	7484	N	JB 336
Noracymethadol	9633		
Norlevorphanol	9634		
Normethadone	9635		Phenyldimazone
Normorphine	9313		
Norpipanone	9636		
Para-Fluorofentanyl	9812		China White, fentanyl
Parahexyl	7374	N	Synhexyl
Peyote	7415	N	Cactus that contains mescaline
Phenadoxone	9637		
Phenampromide	9638		
Phenomorphan	9647		
Phenoperidine	9641		Operidine, Lealgin
Pholcodine	9314		Copholco, Adaphol, Codisol, Lantuss, Pholcolin
Piritramide	9642		Piridolan
Proheptazine	9643		
Properidine	9644		
Propiram	9649		Algeril
Psilocybin	7437	N	Constituent of "magic mushrooms"
Psilocyn	7438	N	Psilocin, constituent of "magic mushrooms"

SCHEDULE I—CONT'D

Substance	DEA Number	Non-narcotic	Other Names
Racemoramide	9645		
Tetrahydrocannabinols	7370	N	THC, Delta-8 THC, Delta-9 THC, and others
Thebacon	9315		Acetylhydrocodone, Acedicon, Thebacetyl
Thiofentanyl	9835		China White, fentanyl
Tilidine	9750		Tilidate, Valoron, Kitadol, Lak, Tilsa
Trimeperidine	9646		Promedolum

SCHEDULE II

Substance	DEA Number	Non-narcotic	Other Names
1-Phenylcyclohexylamine	7460	N	Precursor of PCP
1-Piperidinocyclohexanecarbonitrile	8603	N	PCC, precursor of PCP
Alfentanil	9737		Alfenta
Alphaprodine	9010		Nisentil
Amobarbital	2125	N	Amytal, Tuinal
Amphetamine	1100	N	Dexedrine, Biphetamine
Anileridine	9020		Leritine
Benzoylecgonine	9180		Cocaine metabolite
Bezitramide	9800		Burgodin
Carfentanil	9743		Wildnil
Coca leaves	9040		
Cocaine	9041		Methyl benzoylecgonine, "crack"
Codeine	9050		Morphine methyl ester, methyl morphine
Dextropropoxyphene, bulk (nondosage forms)	9273		Propoxyphene
Dihydrocodeine	9120		Didrate, Parzone
Diphenoxylate	9170		
Diprenorphine	9058		M50-50
Ecgonine	9180		Cocaine precursor, in coca leaves
Ethylmorphine	9190		Dionin
Etorphine HCl	9059		M 99
Fentanyl	9801		Innovar, Sublimaze, Duragesic
Glutethimide	2550	N	Doriden, Dorimide
Hydrocodone	9193		Dihydrocodeinone
Hydromorphone	9150		Dilaudid, dihydromorphinone
Isomethadone	9226		Isoamidone
Levo-alphacetylmethadol	9648		LAAM, long-acting methadone, levomethadyl acetate
Levomethorphan	9210		
Levorphanol	9220		Levo-Dromoran
Meperidine	9230		Demerol, Mepergan, pethidine

(Continued)

SCHEDULE II—CONT'D

Substance	DEA Number	Non-narcotic	Other Names
Meperidine intermediate-A	9232		Meperidine precursor
Meperidine intermediate-B	9233		Meperidine precursor
Meperidine intermediate-C	9234		Meperidine precursor
Metazocine	9240		
Methadone	9250		Dolophine, Methadose, Amidone
Methadone intermediate	9254		Methadone precursor
Methamphetamine	1105	N	Desoxyn, D-desoxyephedrine, ICE, "crank," "speed"
Methylphenidate	1724	N	Ritalin
Metopon	9260		
Moramide-intermediate	9802		
Morphine	9300		MS Contin, Roxanol, Duramorph, RMS, MSIR
Nabilone	7379	N	Cesamet
Opium extracts	9610		
Opium fluid extract	9620		
Opium poppy	9650		Papaver somniferum
Opium tincture	9630		Laudanum
Opium, granulated	9640		Granulated opium
Opium, powdered	9639		Powdered opium
Opium, raw	9600		Raw opium, gum opium
Oxycodone	9143		OxyContin, Percocet, Tylox, Roxicodone, Roxicet,
Oxymorphone	9652		Numorphan
Pentobarbital	2270	N	Nembutal
Phenazocine	9715		Narphen, Prinadol
Phencyclidine	7471	N	PCP, Sernylan
Phenmetrazine	1631	N	Preludin
Phenylacetone	8501	N	P2P, phenyl-2-propanone, benzylmethyl ketone
Piminodine	9730		
Poppy straw	9650		Opium poppy capsules, poppy heads
Poppy straw Concentrate	9670		Concentrate of poppy straw, CPS
Racemethorphan	9732		
Racemorphan	9733		Dromoran
Remifentanil	9739		Ultiva
Secobarbital	2315	N	Seconal, Tuinal
Sufentanil	9740		Sufenta
Thebaine	9333		Precursor of many narcotics

SCHEDULE III

Substance	DEA Number	Non-narcotic	Other Names
Amobarbital and noncontrolled active ingredients	2126	N	Amobarbital/ephedrine capsules
Amobarbital suppository dosage form	2126	N	

SCHEDULE III—CONT'D

Substance	DEA Number	Non-narcotic	Other Names
Anabolic steroids	4000	N	"Body building" drugs
Aprobarbital	2100	N	Alurate
Barbituric acid derivative	2100	N	Barbiturates not specifically listed
Benzphetamine	1228	N	Didrex, Inapetyl
Boldenone	4000	N	Equipoise, Parenabol, Vebonol, dehydrotestosterone
Buprenorphine	9064		Buprenex, Temgesic
Butabarbital	2100	N	Butisol, Butibel
Butalbital	2100	N	Fiorinal, Butalbital with aspirin
Chlorhexadol	2510	N	Mechloral, Mecoral, Medodorm, Chloralodol
Chlorotestosterone (same as clostebol)	4000	N	If 4-chlorotestosterone then clostebol
Chlorphentermine	1645	N	Pre-Sate, Lucofen, Apsedon, Desopimon
Clortermine	1647	N	Voranil
Clostebol	4000	N	Alfa-Trofodermin, Clostene, 4-chlorotestosterone
Codeine and isoquinoline alkaloid 90 mg/du	9803		Codeine with papaverine or noscapine
Codeine combination product 90 mg/du	9804		Empirin, Fiorinal, Tylenol, ASA or APAP w/codeine
Dehydrochlormethyltestosterone	4000	N	Oral-Turinabol
Dihydrocodeine combination product 90 mg/du	9807		Synalgos DC, Compal
Dihydrotestosterone (same as stanolone)	4000	N	See stanolone
Dronabinol in sesame oil in soft gelatin capsule	7369	N	Marinol, synthetic THC in sesame oil/soft gelatin
Drostanolone	4000	N	Drolban, Masterid, Permastril
Ethylestrenol	4000	N	Maxibolin, Orabolin, Durabolin-O, Duraboral
Ethylmorphine combination product 15 mg/du	9808		
Fluoxymesterone	4000	N	Anadroid-F, Halotestin, Ora-Testryl
Formebolone (incorrect spelling in law)	4000	N	Esiclene, Hubernol
Hydrocodone and isoquinoline alkaloid 15 mg/du	9805		Dihydrocodeinone + papaverine or noscapine
Hydrocodone combination product 15 mg/du	9806		Tussionex, Tussend, Lortab, Vicodin, Hycodan, Anexsia ++
Ketamine	7285	N	Ketaset, Ketalar, Special K, K
Lysergic acid	7300	N	LSD precursor
Lysergic acid amide	7310	N	LSD precursor
Mesterolone	4000	N	Proviron

(Continued)

SCHEDULE III—CONT'D

Substance	DEA Number	Non-narcotic	Other Names
Methandienone (see Methandrostenolone)	4000	N	
Methandranone	4000	N	Incorrect spelling of methandienone?
Methandriol	4000	N	Sinesex, Stenediol, Troformone
Methandrostenolone	4000	N	Dianabol, Metabolina, Nerobol, Perbolin
Methenolone	4000	N	Primobolan, Primobolan Depot, Primobolan S
Methyltestosterone	4000	N	Android, Oreton, Testred, Virilon
Methyprylon	2575	N	Noludar
Mibolerone	4000	N	Cheque
Morphine combination product/ 50 mg/100 mL or 100 g	9810		
Nalorphine	9400		Nalline
Nandrolone	4000	N	Deca-Durabolin, Durabolin, Durabolin-50
Norethandrolone	4000	N	Nilevar, Solevar
Opium combination product 25 mg/du	9809		Paregoric, other combination products
Oxandrolone	4000	N	Anavar, Lonavar, Provitar, Vasorome
Oxymesterone	4000	N	Anamidol, Balnimax, Oranabol, Oranabol 10
Oxymetholone	4000	N	Anadrol-50, Adroyd, Anapolon, Anasteron, Pardroyd
Pentobarbital and noncontrolled active ingredients	2271	N	FP-3
Pentobarbital suppository dosage form	2271	N	WANS
Phendimetrazine	1615	N	Plegine, Prelu-2, Bontril, Melfiat, Statobex
Secobarbital and noncontrolled active ingredients	2316	N	Various
Secobarbital suppository dosage form	2316	N	Various
Stanolone	4000	N	Anabolex, Andractim, Pesomax, dihydrotestosterone
Stanozolol	4000	N	Winstrol, Winstrol-V
Stimulant compounds previously excepted	1405	N	Mediatric
Sulfondiethylmethane	2600	N	
Sulfonethylmethane	2605	N	
Sulfonmethane	2610	N	
Talbutal	2100	N	Lotusate

SCHEDULE III—CONT'D

Substance	DEA Number	Non-narcotic	Other Names
Testolactone	4000	N	Teslac
Testosterone	4000	N	Android-T, Androlan, Depotest, Delatestryl
Thiamylal	2100	N	Surital
Thiopental	2100	N	Pentothal
Tiletamine and zolazepam combination product	7295	N	Telazol
Trenbolone	4000	N	Finaplix-S, Finajet, Parabolan
Vinbarbital	2100	N	Delvinal, vinbarbitone

SCHEDULE IV

Substance	DEA Number	Non-narcotic	Other Names
Alprazolam	2882	N	Xanax
Barbital	2145	N	Veronal, Plexonal, barbitone
Bromazepam	2748	N	Lexotan, Lexatin, Lexotanil
Butorphanol	9720	N	Stadol, Stadol NS, Torbugesic, Torbutrol
Camazepam	2749	N	Albego, Limpidon, Paxor
Cathine	1230	N	Constituent of Khat plant
Chloral betaine	2460	N	Beta Chlor
Chloral hydrate	2465	N	Noctec
Chlordiazepoxide	2744	N	Librium, Libritabs, Limbitrol, SK-Lygen
Clobazam	2751	N	Urbadan, Urbanyl
Clonazepam	2737	N	Klonopin, Clonopin
Clorazepate	2768	N	Tranxene
Clotiazepam	2752	N	Trecalmo, Rize
Cloxazolam	2753	N	Enadel, Sepazon, Tolestan
Delorazepam	2754	N	
Dexfenfluramine	1670	N	Redux
Dextropropoxyphene dosage forms	9278		Darvon, propoxyphene, Darvocet, Dolene, Propacet
Diazepam	2765	N	Valium, Valrelease
Dichloralphenazone	2467	N	Midrin, dichloralantipyrine
Diethylpropion	1610	N	Tenuate, Tepanil
Difenoxin 1 mg/25 µg AtSO4/du	9167		Motofen
Estazolam	2756	N	ProSom, Domnamid, Eurodin, Nuctalon
Ethchlorvynol	2540	N	Placidyl
Ethinamate	2545	N	Valmid, Valamin
Ethyl loflazepate	2758	N	
Fencamfamin	1760	N	Reactivan
Fenfluramine	1670	N	Pondimin, Ponderal
Fenproporex	1575	N	Gacilin, Solvolip
Fludiazepam	2759	N	
Flunitrazepam	2763	N	Rohypnol, Narcozep, Darkene, Roipnol
Flurazepam	2767	N	Dalmane
Halazepam	2762	N	Paxipam

(Continued)

SCHEDULE IV—CONT'D

Substance	DEA Number	Non-narcotic	Other Names
Haloxazolam	2771	N	
Ketazolam	2772	N	Anxon, Loftran, Solatran, Contamex
Loprazolam	2773	N	
Lorazepam	2885	N	Ativan
Lormetazepam	2774	N	Noctamid
Mazindol	1605	N	Sanorex, Mazanor
Mebutamate	2800	N	Capla
Medazepam	2836	N	Nobrium
Mefenorex	1580	N	Anorexic, Amexate, Doracil, Pondinil
Meprobamate	2820	N	Miltown, Equanil, Deprol, Equagesic, Meprospan
Methohexital	2264	N	Brevital
Methylphenobarbital (mephobarbital)	2250	N	Mebaral, mephobarbital
Midazolam	2884	N	Versed
Modafinil	1680	N	Provigil
Nimetazepam	2837	N	Erimin
Nitrazepam	2834	N	Mogadon
Nordiazepam	2838	N	Nordazepam, Demadar, Madar
Oxazepam	2835	N	Serax, Serenid-D
Oxazolam	2839	N	Serenal, Convertal
Paraldehyde	2585	N	Paral
Pemoline	1530	N	Cylert
Pentazocine	9709	N	Talwin, Talwin NX, Talacen, Talwin compound
Petrichloral	2591	N	Pentaerythritol chloral, Periclor
Phenobarbital	2285	N	Luminal, Donnatal, Bellergal-S
Phentermine	1640	N	Ionamin, Fastin, Adipex-P, Obe-Nix, Zantryl
Pinazepam	2883	N	Domar
Pipradrol	1750	N	Detaril, Stimolag Fortis
Prazepam	2764	N	Centrax
Quazepam	2881	N	Doral, Dormalin
Sibutramine	1675	N	Meridia
SPA	1635	N	1-dimethylamino-1,2-diphenylethane, Lefetamine
Temazepam	2925	N	Restoril
Tetrazepam	2886	N	
Triazolam	2887	N	Halcion
Zaleplon	2781	N	Sonata
Zolpidem	2783	N	Ambien, Stilnoct, Ivadal

SCHEDULE V

Codeine preparations: 200 mg/100 mL or 100 g			Cosanyl, Robitussin A-C, Cheracol, Cerose, Pediacof

SCHEDULE V—CONT'D

Substance	DEA Number	Non-narcotic	Other Names
Difenoxin preparations: 0.5 mg/25 µg AtSO4/du			Motofen
Dihydrocodeine preparations: 10 mg/100 mL or 100 g			Cophene-S, various others
Diphenoxylate preparations: 2.5 mg/25 µg AtSO4			Lomotil, Logen
Ethylmorphine preparations: 100 mg/100 mL or 100 g			
Opium preparations: 100 mg/100 mL or 100 g			Parepectolin, Kapectolin PG, Kaolin Pectin P.G.
Pyrovalerone	1485	N	Centroton, Thymergix

U.S. Drug Enforcement Administration (DEA): Drug Scheduling. Available at http://www.usdoj.gov/dea/pubs/scheduling.html.

Index

Page numbers followed by f indicate figures; t, tables; b, boxes.